BOSCH REVOLUTION
MUSCLES MADE TO MOVE

By Greg Bosch

Copyright © GREG BOSCH, 2023 ALL RIGHTS RESERVED.

This Book teaches the effective use of the Trigger Point Release Tool product of Bosch Activation, LLC. Photo CREDITS, Logo and Cover Image,

Bosch Activation, LLC.

Child Soccer Player, Photo by Pollyana Ventura on Getty Images

Running Athlete, Photo by SHOTPRIME on CANSTOCKPHOTO

Reference Books and Magnifying Glass, Photo by Mark Wragg on Getty Images/iStock
Tennis Player Sport Recreation (Back Cover Image), Photo by Bobex-73 on iStock
Cardio Gym Training, Photo by Stefan Dalh on Dreamstime

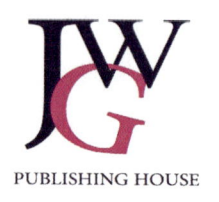

JWG
PUBLISHING HOUSE

BOSCH REVOLUTION

This book is dedicated to God from whom all blessings flow. Thank you for allowing me to serve you. I am grateful to Aaron Mattes my mentor, for teaching me Active Isolated Stretching and Strengthening (AIS). I would like to recognize my Mom and Dad for their love and support over the years—as well as my brother, Mike Bosch, and my sister, Susan Nyman. I have had unwavering support from Vincent & Pam Marino and Anthony Marino. Key people in my photos that helped make this book are Oliver Crawford, Pro Tennis Player ATP #203, Carson Baker, a Tennis player at the University of Mississippi. Marianna Singletary, Volleyball Player at the University of Texas, 2023 NCAA National Champions.

I would also like to recognize my friends, Dan Totman, a physiotherapist in Columbus, OH, and Rick Carlisle, the Head Coach of the Indiana Pacers.

I want to thank my cousin, Kate Gorski, for editing this book.

CONTENTS

Introduction 7
Understanding injury proneness 8
Trigger Points 11
Releasing Fascia 13
Introducing The Trigger point release Tool™ 14
 benefits of using the TPRT 17
   For Therapists 17
   For Clients 17
Contraindications 19
Preparing to Use the tprt 20
   Self-Massage: Preparing for use of TPRT 20
   Therapist or Athletic Trainer: Preparing a Client for a TRPT Session 20
TPRT MODULE 1 – SELF THERAPY 21
   QUAD #1 – CURVE POINT 1 & POINT 2 22
   QUAD #2 (LUBRICATION) – CURVE POINT 1 & POINT 2 23
   INSIDE HAMSTRING – CURVE 24
   OUTSIDE HAMSTRING – CURVE 25
   IT BAND – SLOPE AND FLAT EDGE 26
   ADDUCTOR - INSIDE LEG - CURVE, POINT 1 & POINT 2 27
   FRONT CALF - CURVE & POINT 28
   FRONT CALF – PIN & ROCK - CURVE & POINT 1 OR 2 29
   QUAD – PIN & ROCK - POINT 1 & CURVE 30
   QUAD (INSIDE) PIN & RELEASE – CURVE & POINT 1 31
   QUAD (OUTSIDE) - INSIDE POINT 1 32
   MEDIAL (INSIDE QUAD) – PIN & ROCK - POINT 2 33
   BACK (POSTERIOR) CALF - CURVES 34
   LOW BACK OVER SHIRT– POINT 1 & 2 35
   ABS – FLAT EDGE OVER SHIRT 36
   OUTSIDE ABS – FLAT EDGE OVER SHIRT 37
   MEDIAL (INSIDE) FOREARM – SMALL KNOB 38
   AB RELEASE (SUPINE 1) – SLOPE 40

AB RELEASE (SUPINE 2) – SLOPE 41

ILIACUS RELEASE – SMALL KNOB 42

PSOAS DISTAL ATTACHMENT (SIDE LYING) – SMALL KNOB 43

AB RELEASE (STANDING): RECTUS ABDOMINUS - SLOPES 44

TPRT™ MODULE 3 – Client Therapy 45

FOREARM 45

FOREARM – SLOPE 46

ANTERIOR FOREARM (SIDE LYING)–CURVE, SLOPE, FLAT EDGE 47

ANTERIOR FOREARM (SIDE LYING)–CURVE, SLOPE, FLAT EDGE 48

ANTERIOR FOREARM (SUPINE) – CURVE 49

TPRT™ MODULE 4 – Client Therapy 50

ARM RELEASE (SIDE LYING AND PRONE) - FLAT EDGE 51

ARM RELEASE: MIDDLE BICEPS BRACHII - CURVE AND SLOPE 52

DISTAL BICEPS RELEASE - CURVE 53

POSTERIOR ROTATOR CUFF & TRICEPS 54

TRICEPS AND SERRATUS ANTERIOR RELEASE – CURVE & SMALL KNOB 55

TRICEPS RELEASE (PRONE) - CURVE 56

SHOULDER RELEASE (PRONE) - CURVE 57

TPRT™ MODULE 5 – Client Therapy 58

FOOT RELEASE PART 1 - SMALL KNOB 58

FOOT RELEASE PART 2 - SMALL KNOB 59

FOOT RELEASE PART 1 & 2 - SLOPE AND FLAT EDGE 60

MEDIAL (INSIDE) CALF RELEASE - CURVE 61

LATERAL (OUTSIDE) CALF RELEASE PART 1 - CURVE 62

LATERAL (OUTSIDE) CALF RELEASE PART 2 - CURVE 63

CALF RELEASE: GASTROC (PRONE) – V & CURVES 64

HOW TO RELEASE THE CALF (PRONE) 65

TPRT™ MODULE 6 – Client Therapy 66

QUAD RELEASE - ABOVE KNEE (SEATED) – SLOPE, V & CURVES 66

IT BAND AND QUAD RELEASE (SEATED) – SLOPE, V & CURVES 67

PATELLA RELEASE (SEATED) 68

IT BAND RELEASE (SIDE LYING) PART 1 –CURVE 69

IT BAND RELEASE (SIDE LYING) PART 2 –CURVES 70

ADDUCTOR RELEASE (INNER THIGH) – SLOPE & CURVE 71

- PSOAS RELEASE 72
- HAMSTRING RELEASE (PRONE) – SLOPE & FLAT EDGE 73
- HAMSTRING RELEASE (PRONE/SIDE-LYING) - SMALL KNOB 74

TPRT™ MODULE 7 – Client Therapy 75

- GLUTE MAX (PRONE) – CURVE 75
- GLUTE MEDIUS RELEASE - SMALL KNOB 76
- GLUTE MEDIUS RELEASE (SIDE LYING) - SMALL KNOB & CURVE 77
- INTERNAL ROTATION ASSESSMENT - TFL RELEASE SMALL KNOB 78
- HIP EXTERNAL ROTATORS- QUADRATUS FEMORIS – SMALL KNOB & FLAT EDGE 79
- QUADRATUS LUMBORUM (SIDELYING) – V & CURVES 80
- LATISSIMUS DORSI (PRONE) – SLOPE & CURVE 81
- BACK RELEASE (PRONE) - SMALL KNOB 82
- BACK RELEASE (SEATED) - SMALL KNOB 83
- TRAP RELEASE (SEATED) - CURVE 84
- LOWER BACK RELEASE (STANDING) - CURVE 85
- RECTUS ABDOMINIS AND INTERNAL OBLIQUE RELEASE – SLOPE 86

Conclusion 87

Meet the Author 89

- SOME OF GREG'S CLIENTS 89

INTRODUCTION

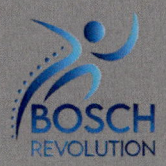

Understanding and addressing injury proneness is a topic widely discussed in the fields of athletics and general physical fitness and well-being. It is also of great interest to those concerned with maintaining optimal health as they age. We know that an exercise regimen is essential for optimal health and avoiding injury. But your muscles must be prepared for safe, effective strength training.

In Muscles Made to Move, I will share my therapy tools to prepare your muscles, fascia, and nerves so you can train/exercise more safely and efficiently and minimize muscle fatigue and soreness. In this book, you will learn how to use my Trigger Point Release Tool™ (TPRT™) to help you loosen fascia restrictions and prepare your muscles for strength training and recovery.

Many athletes and weekend warriors have a different mindset than the everyday person. They want to push their body to the limits of their strength and endurance. This puts too much strain on muscles and tension on joints, leading to injuries. This overtraining causes lactic acid waste buildup in your muscles. When muscles become short and tight, the fascia will stick and adhere to the muscle, causing you to lose flexibility, strength, and power. Muscles Made to Move will teach you how to care for your muscles so they become more pliable and flexible, enabling you to move your joints through their full range of motion.

UNDERSTANDING INJURY PRONENESS

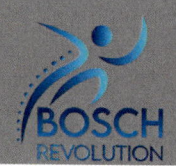

The concept of being injury-prone raises questions about its causes and potential solutions. Whether you've observed it in athletes or experienced it yourself, understanding the factors contributing to injury proneness is crucial. This book explores preventative ways to avoid injuries and the management and solution for injuries by introducing training techniques and the Trigger Point Release Tool™.

Injury-Prone is described as "frequently injured or often sustaining injuries." It encompasses a range of injuries, from constant minor sprains to more severe incidents like a ruptured Achilles tendon. The term is not limited to only professional athletes; recreational athletes may also face injury concerns. Two types of injuries, acute and overuse, contribute to the overall understanding of injury proneness.

Studies involving coaches, trainers, physical therapists, and doctors have identified three main factors responsible for injuries:

1. Overtraining
2. Incorrect sports techniques
3. Physiological or anatomical factors

According to one functional neurologist, Garrett Salpeter, "Inefficiency in movement mechanics plays a significant role in injury proneness. When muscles lack proper elongation, force absorption during deceleration becomes compromised, potentially leading to issues in connective tissue and bones."

Understanding movement mechanics is crucial for preventing injuries. Athletes, both professional and recreational, often rely on habitual movements that, if not aligned with proper technique, can result in micro-tears or fractures. Failure to correct these issues may escalate into more severe injuries over time. Addressing movement mechanics is essential for injury prevention, and rehabilitation often employs this principle.

Some genetic predispositions have been identified as influential in injury risk. Specific variations in the COL1A1 gene, responsible for collagen production in tendons and ligaments, have been linked to soft tissue injuries.

Genetic testing can provide valuable insights for athletes, helping them understand and mitigate their injury risks.

UNDERSTANDING INJURY PRONENESS

Another risk is soft tissue injuries, which affect – muscles, tendons, ligaments, and nerves. Genetic factors influence these injuries. Variations in the COL1A1 gene have been associated with ACL injuries, Achilles tendon ruptures, and shoulder dislocations. Also, genes impact muscle fatigue, influencing how quickly lactate is cleared from muscle cells.

Genetic variations, such as those in the MCT1 gene, affect muscle fatigue by influencing lactate clearance. Genetics also influences post-exercise recovery, impacting the body's response to oxidative stress and inflammation. Understanding these genetic aspects helps tailor training and recovery strategies.

While injury proneness is a complex interplay of genetics, movement mechanics, and training habits, awareness and proactive measures can significantly reduce the risk of sports injuries. Whether you're a professional athlete or a recreational enthusiast, understanding your genetic predispositions and adopting appropriate training practices can enhance performance and minimize the impact of injuries.

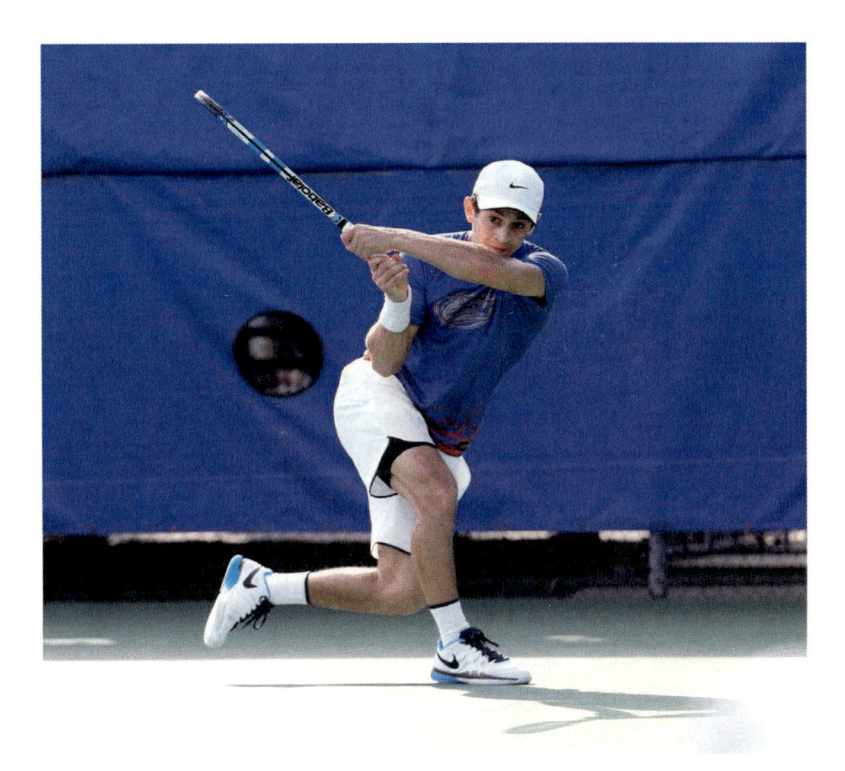

Elliot Orkin – Tennis player who went to the University of Florida and worked with Greg.

Greg Bosch, 2023, All rights reserved.

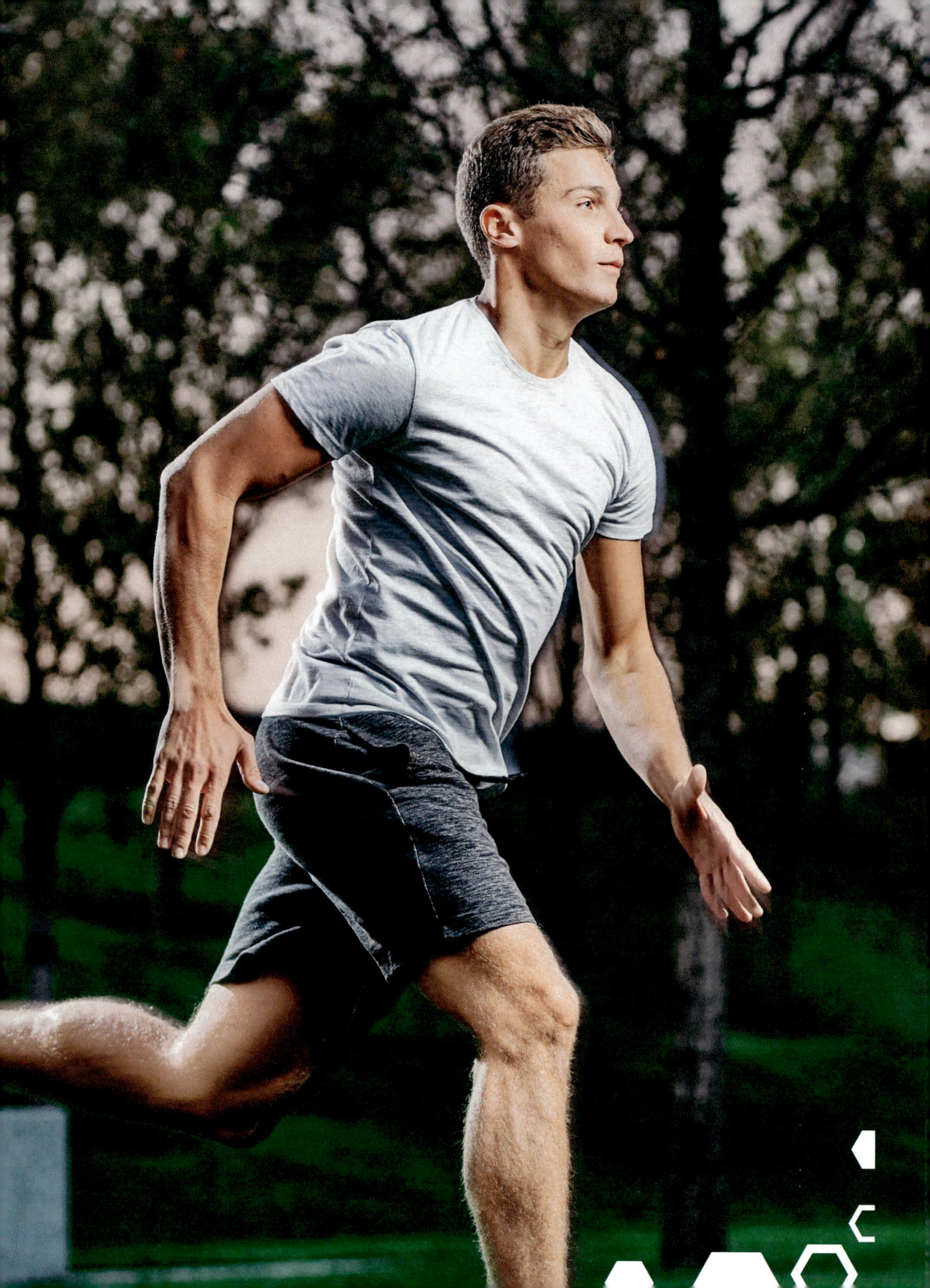

TRIGGER POINTS

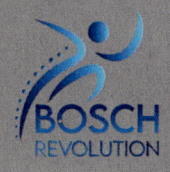

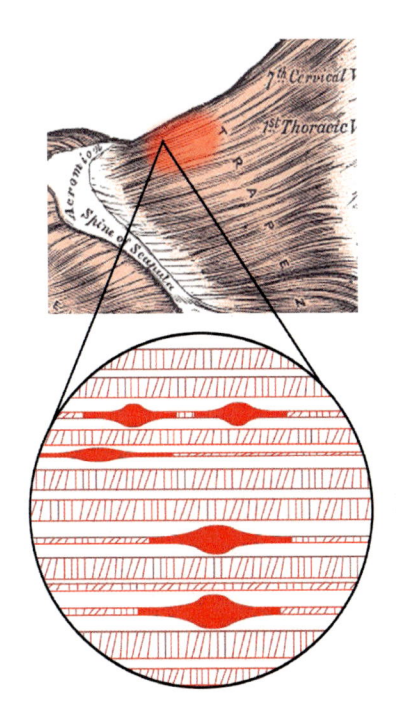

A trigger point develops when sensory nerves become sensitized within a taut band of muscle, causing the generation of local and referred pain upon compression.

The underlying cause of a taut band is a hyperactive motor nerve branch. This branch generates sustained contractions in the muscle fibers it supplies, specifically those attached to the motor endplate.

When a portion of the muscle experiences sustained contraction (forming the taut band), it compresses the blood vessels within that area.

https://upload.wikimedia.org/wikipedia/commons/f/f2/Trigger_Point_Complex.jpg https://ostrowonline.usc.edu/trigger-point-mapping

This reduced blood flow leads to the accumulation of metabolic by-products resulting from the muscle's contraction.

The presence of these metabolic waste products further aggravates and sensitizes the sensory nerve fibers located nearest to the hyperactive motor endplate. These nerves, known as Type IV or C-fibers, exhibit tenderness to pressure (mechanical allodynia) and may cause spontaneous pain.

As these sensory nerve fibers fire spontaneously, they initiate a process known as central sensitization. This involves the sensitization of the 2nd order neuron in the brain stem or spinal cord, which, when strongly stimulated, can result in referred pain.

TRIGGER POINTS

Trigger points develop because of muscular injuries, strains, and trauma. Small tears can occur in the associated soft tissues when muscle fibers, fascia, ligaments, or tendons are weakened, overstretched, or inflamed. As the tissue heals, it contracts and becomes twisted and knotted. These knotted fibers restrict the fresh blood supply necessary for the muscle cells.

Additionally, muscle fibers often shorten to protect themselves from further injury. The Trigger Point Release Tool (TPRT™) is designed to address these issues effectively. (Please refer to the Contour Page to learn more about this tool's features, including its Flat Edge and Slopes.)

Trigger points often form in injured muscles, which are an excellent place to look for them.

An active trigger point is painful when palpated and produces referred pain when squeezed. A latent trigger point is not painful and produces referred pain when squeezed.

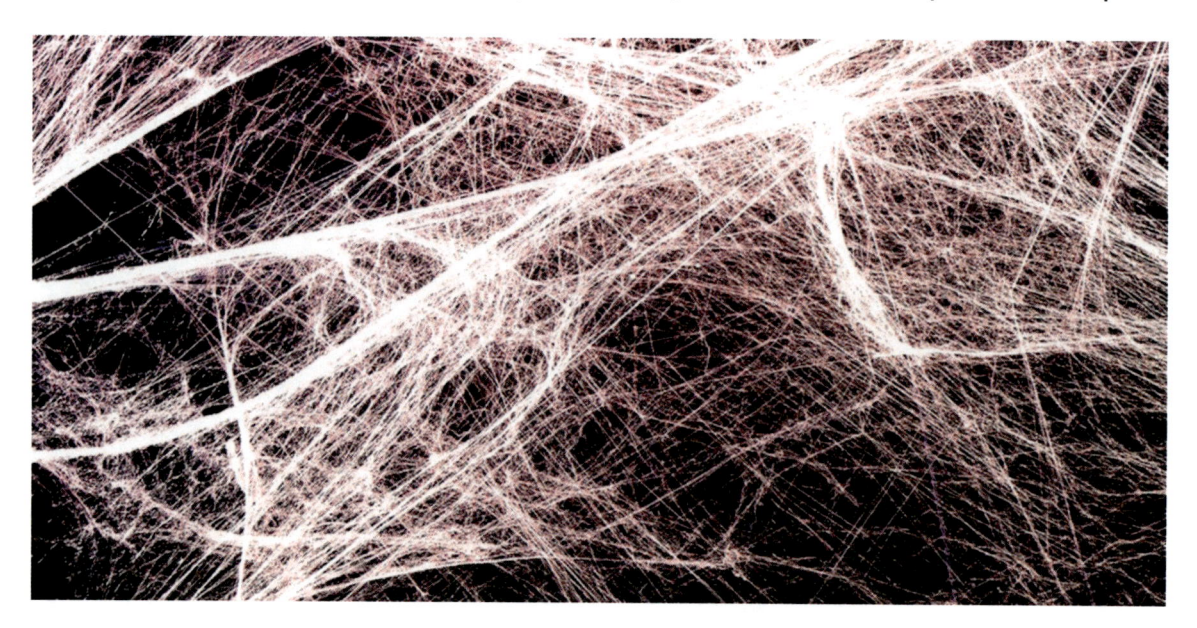

The Intricate Web of Fascia

https://kinetik-fitness.com/wp-content/uploads/2018/03/download-5.jpg

RELEASING FASCIA

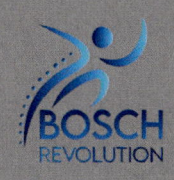

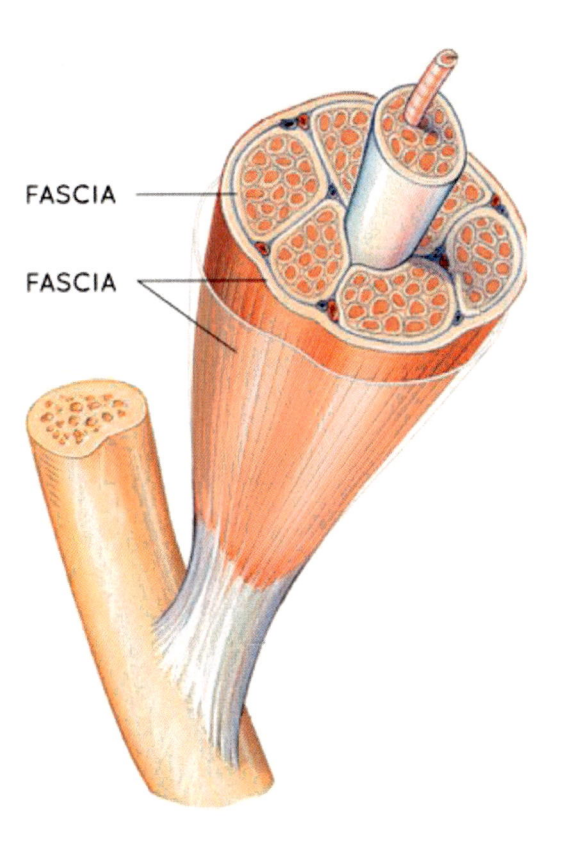

FASCIA

FASCIA

"Fascia is a thin sheath of fibrous tissue enclosing muscles or other organs. An easier way to visualize how fascia works in our bodies is to think of it as an intricate web.

Our fascial system is uninterrupted as a web and runs from head to toe. This dense tissue covers every muscle, bone, nerve, and other soft tissue in the body, including our organs, arteries, and veins.

Our fascia is essentially responsible for holding our bodies together."

https://www.marquettept.com/2018/11/27/what-is-fascia-and-how-does-it- contribute-to-pain/

Here is a list of a few simple techniques that may help with your fascia pain:

- *Hydrate* - This helps keep tissue lubricated and pliable.
- *Move Frequently* - Don't sit in one place for too long, as this can cause fascia and muscles to get stuck in one position.
- *Stretch Gently*—Before you leave bed in the morning, Try stretching your arms and legs out and gently rolling from side to side.
- In this book, you will learn how to use the TPRT to release fascia.
- *Warm Up Before You Exercise* - Walk for 10 minutes.

As fascia mats down to muscles, nerves, and bones, it limits joint and muscle mobility. Releasing fascia is an art, as fascia plays a vital role in our overall health.

INTRODUCING THE TRIGGER POINT RELEASE TOOL™

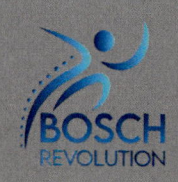

Do you inadvertently train your body for dysfunction? Do you: hold your breath while exercising? Grit your teeth and strain your neck muscles? Raise your shoulder(s) towards your ear(s)? Shift your head to the right or left? Curl your toes?

These are all types of muscle contractions that create patterns of imbalance. They will weaken your posture, balance, and stability if left unattended.

The Bosch Revolution Trigger Point Release Tool™ (TPRT) has scientifically designed Curves and contours to unwind restricted fascia, release tight muscles, and increase blood flow to muscles, flushing out toxins and waste products. It is made of cold rolled steel, and its most important mechanical properties are impact, resistance, and toughness.

This book will teach you how to use the TPRT to improve blood flow and muscle tone, release trigger points, and improve the pliability of your fascia so you can move more easily.

The TPRT:

- Quickly improves recovery times between workouts.

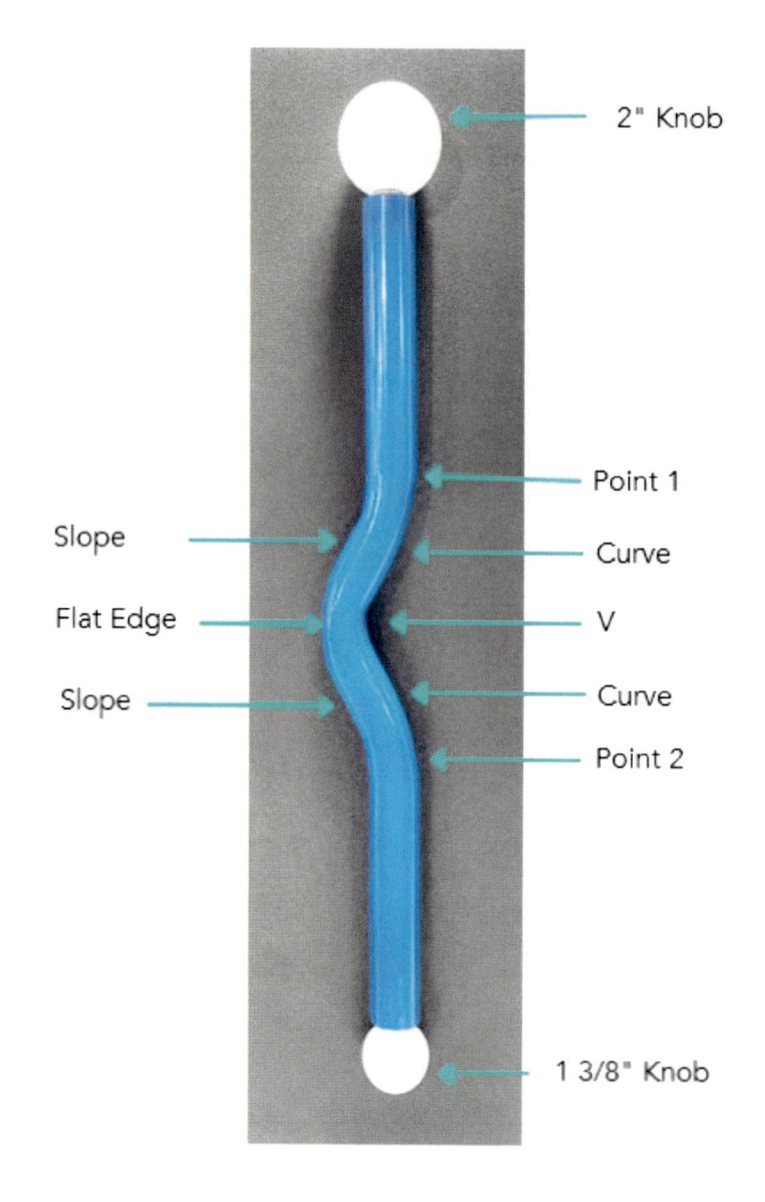

- Prepares muscles and fascia for flexibility and strength training.
- Is easily used between sets when working out.
- Is designed with Curves and Slopes that conform to your muscles, allowing you to free difficult-to-get-at areas where fascia becomes restricted and adheres to muscles.

The Curve is the most forgiving portion of the tool. Using each of the following will increase the pressure, starting with the Flat Edge, Slopes, Points, and Knobs.

You can apply lotion to the skin for smooth, fluid movements or use the TPRT directly over your clothes.

Using the TPRT exponentially increases the effectiveness of one's workout or therapy session.

The TPRT is lightweight and user-friendly. Because of its unique size and shape, the contours and Curves allow the user to reach hard-to-reach muscles and apply more pressure than using their hands. This is great for individual use and saves the hands of massage therapists, physical therapists, athletic trainers, and chiropractors!

For athletes who want cutting-edge training, the TPRT uniquely prepares their bodies for their workout regimen or competition. It also helps to maintain optimal performance during workouts or games and decreases recovery time.

Many people do yoga, pilates, and CrossFit without first preparing their muscles for these activities. If you are sore and stiff after your workouts, adding the TPRT to your pre-and post-workout is important so you can stretch more effectively.

Pre-workout: This allows you to warm the muscles up and frees the fascial restrictions that bind up your joints and limit your mobility. Remember, muscles must be lengthened before they can be properly strengthened.

In between sets: TPRT can be used on big muscles like quads, hamstrings, glutes, and abs to stimulate nerve endings and increase blood flow to fatigued muscles.

Post-workout: The TPRT moves lactic acid into the bloodstream, improving recovery times.

The TPRT can be a more effective alternative to massage therapy guns, which may overstimulate the nerve endings and ultimately weaken the joint. Our body's electrical system is far more delicate than we realize it to be. These overpowering tools can be too intense for the nerves and the muscles.

My goal is to teach you the art of soft tissue release with my TPRT™.

IMPORTANT

This product is not a medical device.

Consult your doctor before beginning any exercise or therapy program.

Read and follow all warnings and information before using this product to reduce any risk of injury.

Always use proper techniques and common sense when exercising or doing therapy. Serious or fatal injury can occur. Exercise and therapy programs of any kind present a possible danger to the participant or recipient.

Before each use, check your equipment for any signs of damage, defects, or wear. If any is found, discontinue use immediately and contact Bosch Revolution for assistance.

All Bosch Revolution Equipment, including the Trigger Point Release Tool™ (TPRT™), are intended to be used by adults only in the manner shown/ illustrated/ described. Anyone under the age of 18 should have constant adult supervision.

BENEFITS OF USING THE TPRT

The TPRT offers numerous benefits to massage therapists and clients (professional athletes, weekend warriors, or everyday people looking to get out of pain).

For Therapists

Massage Therapists, Physical Therapists, Trainers, and Chiropractors

The TPRT saves your hands, allows you to leverage pressure on your clients, helps you access difficult-to-reach muscles around the hips and groin, and establishes your credibility as you demonstrate expertise with soft tissue tools.

For Clients

Professional athletes, weekend warriors, or everyday people who are looking to get out of pain

- Reduces joint inflammation and heart rate. Improves range of motion and flexibility. Breaks up scar tissue around muscles and joints. Improves recovery times.
- Pain relief from headaches.
- Better sleep.
- Higher energy levels.
- Enhances your workout and athletic performance—use TPRT in between sets for quads, abs, lower back, and hamstrings.
- Releases endorphins.
- Decreases muscle spasms and cramps. Improves oxygen flow.
- Decreases blood pressure. Increases hemoglobin production.
- Adds a new skill set to your toolbox.

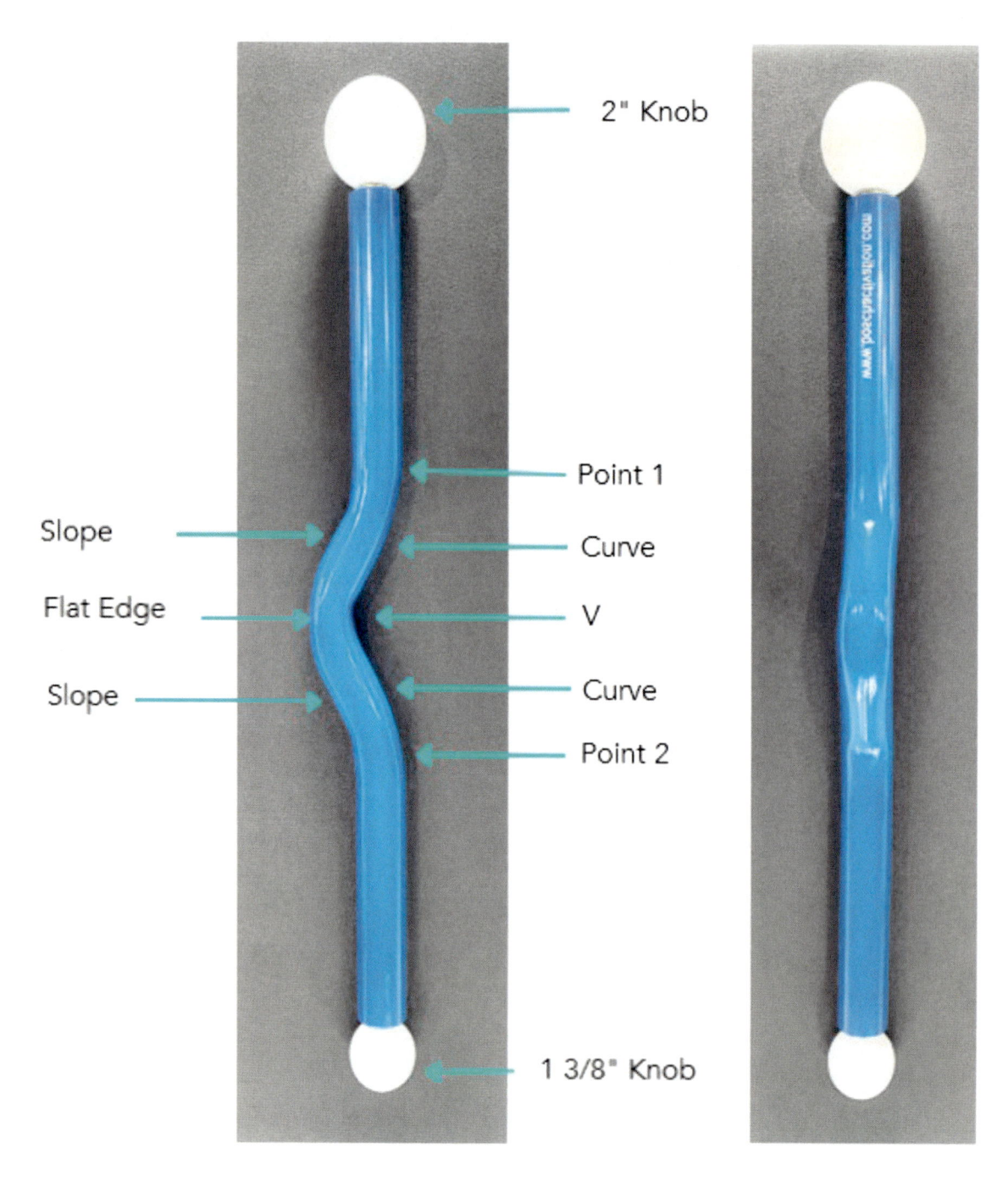

Applications of the TPRT™ can be used:

- To slide over your clothes.
- On the skin with or without lotion.
- To pin and release fascia.
- To slide over muscles (apply lotion to your skin to reduce friction)

CONTRAINDICATIONS

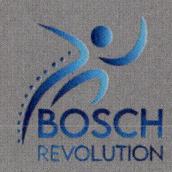

The TPRT is a valuable addition to your massage therapy toolbox. However, certain clients may not benefit from using this instrument. Clients such as older people, infants, children under 12, individuals with low muscle tone regardless of age, or those who simply do not prefer deep tissue work should be considered.

Contraindications are areas on the body you will want to avoid using the Trigger Point Release Tool™ (TPRT).

You should avoid using the TPRT in areas with fractures (broken bones), rashes, contusions, hematomas, bruises, dislocations, poison ivy, open wounds, sunburn, etc. If your skin easily bruises, you should take caution and work very lightly.

PRODUCT LIABILITY INDEMNIFICATION

By using this product, the Buyer agrees to indemnify, defend, and hold harmless the Seller, its Affiliates, and their respective employees, officers, directors, and agents (each referred to as a 'Seller Indemnified Party') from any and all liability, loss, damage, expenses (including reasonable attorney's fees and expenses), and costs (collectively referred to as 'liabilities') that may be incurred by the Seller Indemnified Party as a result of or arising from: By using this product, the Buyer agrees to indemnify, defend, and hold harmless the Seller, its Affiliates, and their respective employees, officers, directors, and agents (each referred to as a 'Seller Indemnified Party') from any and all liability, loss, damage, expenses (including reasonable attorney's fees and expenses), and costs (collectively referred to as 'liabilities') that may be incurred by the Seller Indemnified Party as a result of or arising from:

- (a) personal injury or death of any person caused using the Bosch Revolution Trigger Point Release Tool™ (TPRT) or any product sold by the Buyer, its Affiliates, or its Licensees or sublicensees in relation to pre-clinical or clinical studies conducted by Bosch Revolution LLC for the Trigger Point Release Tool™ (TPRT) or packaging products.

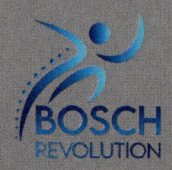

PREPARING TO USE THE TPRT

Self-Massage: Preparing for the use of TPRT

First, determine whether you will work through your clothing or apply lotion or oil to your skin. Wearing sweatpants or tights that don't have pockets is preferable if you are working through clothing. If you use lotion or oil, you will want to wear shorts and a tank top or loose-fitting clothing.

Therapist or Athletic Trainer: Preparing a Client for a TRPT Session

If you are a therapist or athletic trainer working through your client's clothing, have them wear sweatpants or tights that don't have pockets. Likewise, if you choose to use oil or lotion, have your client wear shorts, a tank top, or loose-fitting clothing.

Working through clothing is a different experience from working with lotion or oil directly on the skin. Most lotions will absorb into the skin and dry quickly. You have a short time window to use the TPRT when using lotion. When using oil, you have a longer window of time to slide the tool on the skin. Short, small movements allow you to get deeper into the muscle to release fascia. You can also use small movements when working through clothing, but it has a different effect on the muscles. If you want to do trigger point release techniques around joints, it's better NOT to use lotion or oil. You can use the rubber knobs directly on the skin or through clothing. This allows you to engage the tissues to go deeper or to work in different directions around the joints. Have the client breathe in for three seconds and apply the pressure for 3 to 5 seconds as they exhale.

Release and repeat, applying the pressure on the exhale.

Once you have released the tissues (muscles around the joint) 2 to 3 times, you will move the rubber knob to another area.

TPRT MODULE 1 – SELF THERAPY

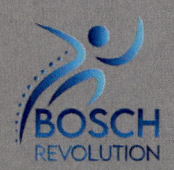

This section is designed for the personal use of the Trigger Point Release Tool by individuals desiring to maintain optimal health no matter their everyday routine. It is used before and after workouts by:

- athletes
- weekend warriors
- people who sit or stand all day or
- people who do heavy lifting, etc.

The following Module addresses releasing the following:

- quads
- hamstrings
- inner thigh
- IT bands
- calves
- lower back
- abs
- forearms

TPRT MODULE 1 – SELF THERAPY

QUAD #1 – CURVE POINT 1 & POINT 2

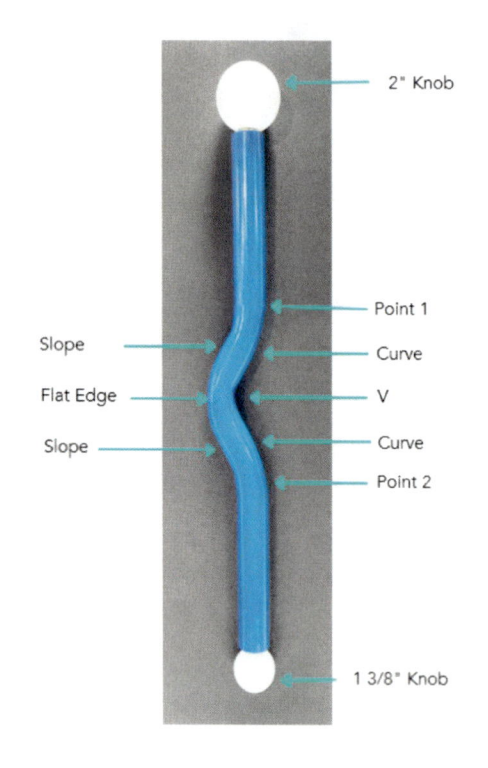

LUBRICATION: None

TPRT:

Use the Curves, V, Points 1 & 2 to apply light pressure with the TPRT.

TECHNIQUE MOTION:

Engage muscle tissue - _Pin and lock down_ on the muscles with moderate pressure, then move tissue side to side, up and down, see-saw motion.

TIME:

15-30 seconds

Quad - Curve - Point 1, & 2

BREATHING TECHNIQUE:

Breathe in for 3 seconds. As you exhale for 5 seconds, apply moderate pressure with the tool and engage the muscles and the tissues by moving the tool side to side and back and forth. Do not slide.

TPRT MODULE 1 – SELF THERAPY

QUAD #2 (LUBRICATION) – CURVE POINT 1 & POINT 2

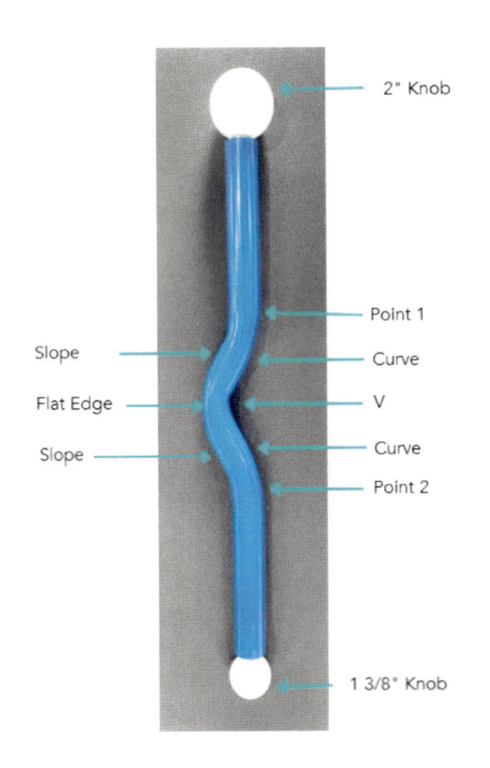

LUBRICATION: Lotion or Oil

TPRT:
Use the Curves, V, Points 1 & 2 to apply light pressure with the TPRT.

TECHNIQUE MOTION:
Apply lotion to the quad. Use the Curves and V to slide the TPRT up and down the quad. Vary speed and pressure. Change angles and pressure by raising the left hand and lowering the right, and vice versa.

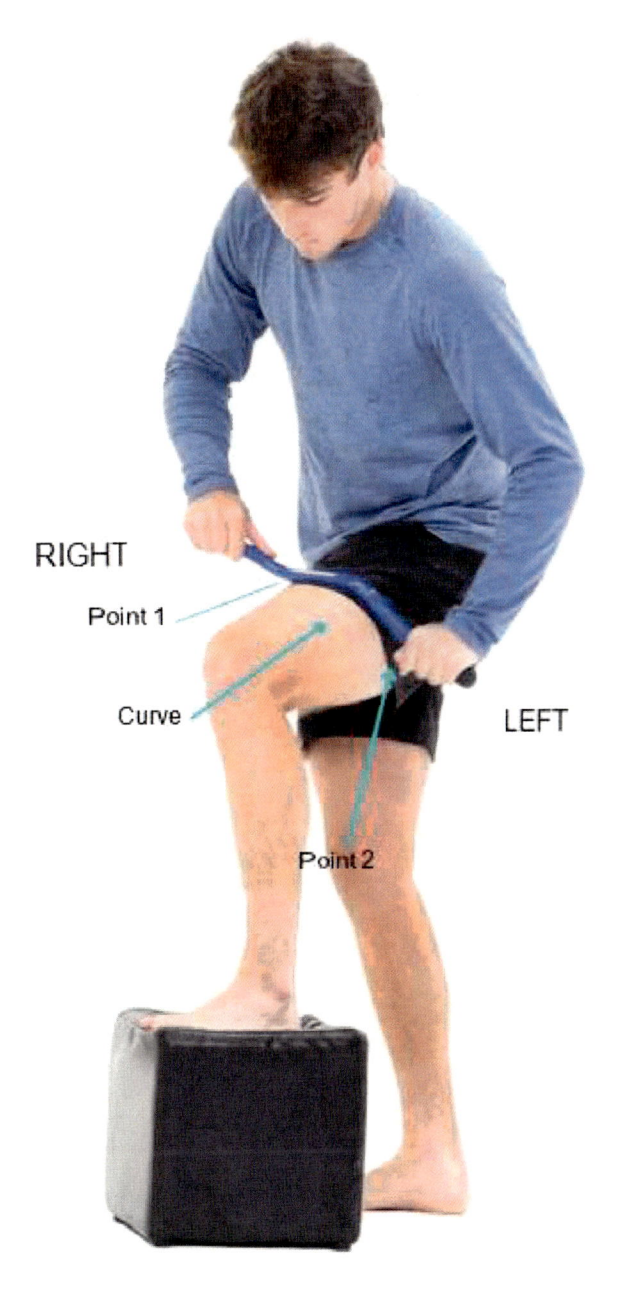

TIME:
15-30 seconds

Quad – Curve - Point 1, & 2

BREATHING TECHNIQUE:

Breathe in for 3 seconds. As you exhale for 5 seconds, apply moderate pressure with the tool and slide up and down the quad. This will allow you to leverage the Curves and the Points.

TPRT MODULE 1 – SELF THERAPY

INSIDE HAMSTRING – CURVE

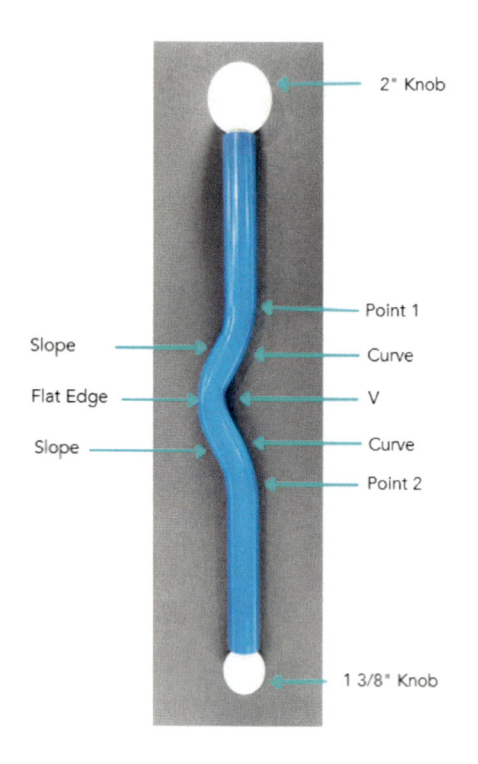

LUBRICATION: None

TPRT:
Use the Curves, V, Points 1 & 2 to apply light and heavy pressure with the TPRT to release trigger points.

TECHNIQUE MOTION:
Use the Curves and V to <u>pivot</u> the TPRT up and down. Change angles and pressure by raising the left hand up and lowering the right and vice versa. This will allow you to use the Curves and the Points for more leverage.

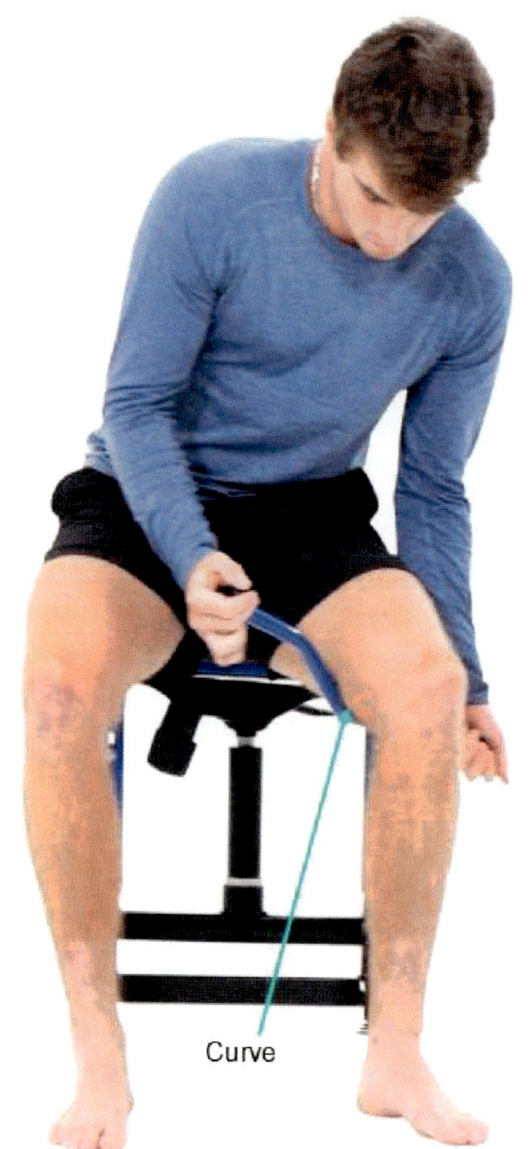

TIME:
15-30 seconds

BREATHING TECHNIQUE:
Breathe in for 3 seconds, and exhale for 5 seconds.

Inside Hamstring - Curve

TPRT MODULE 1 – SELF THERAPY

OUTSIDE HAMSTRING – CURVE

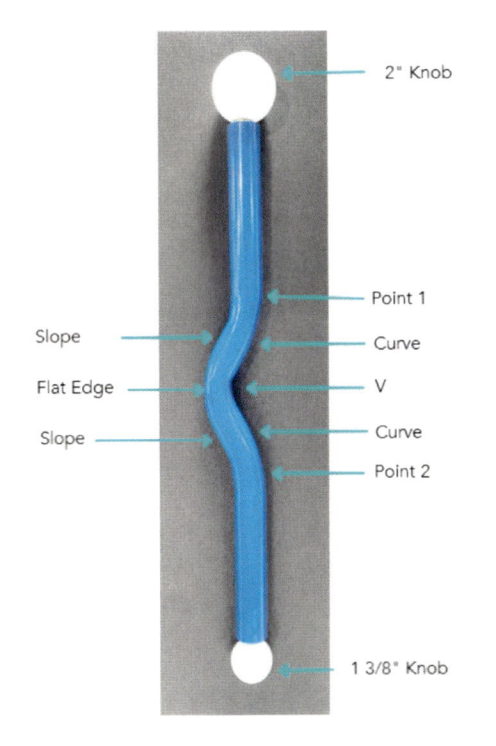

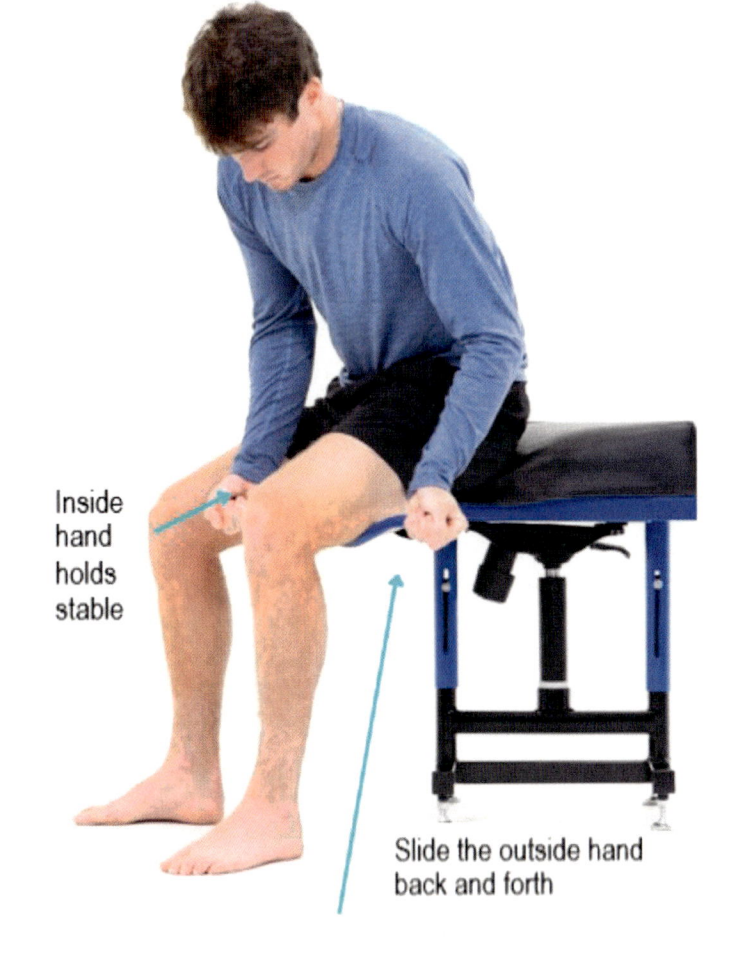

Outside Hamstring - Curve

LUBRICATION: Lotion or Oil

TPRT:
Use the Curve to apply light to heavy pressure with the TPRT to release trigger points.

TECHNIQUE MOTION:
Use the Curve and V to slide the TPRT up and down. The inside hand will hold stable, then raise the left up and slide back and forth. *The right hand will hold stable, then raise the left up and slide back and forth.*

TIME:
15-30 seconds

BREATHING TECHNIQUE:
Breathe in for 3 seconds. As you exhale for 5 seconds, apply moderate pressure with the TPRT.

25

TPRT MODULE 1 – SELF THERAPY

IT BAND – SLOPE AND FLAT EDGE

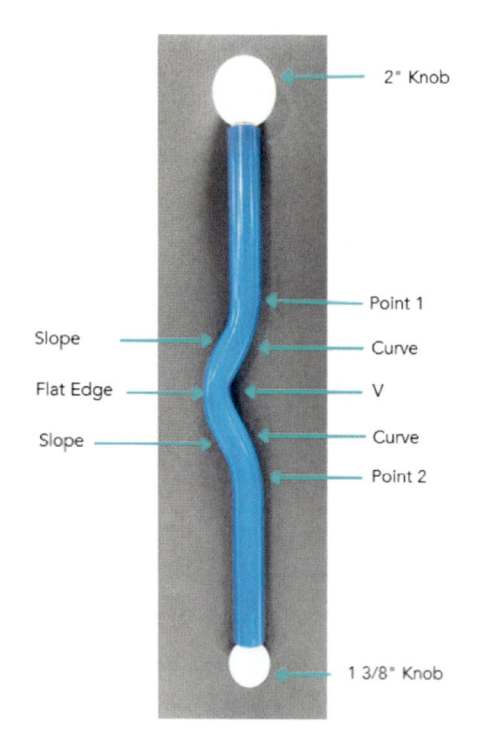

LUBRICATION: Lotion or oil

TPRT:

Use the Slopes and Flat Edges of the TPRT to release trigger points.

TECHNIQUE MOTION:

Use the Slope and Flat Edge to slide the TPRT up and down your IT Band. *Change angles and pressure by raising up the left hand and lowering the right hand, and vice versa.*

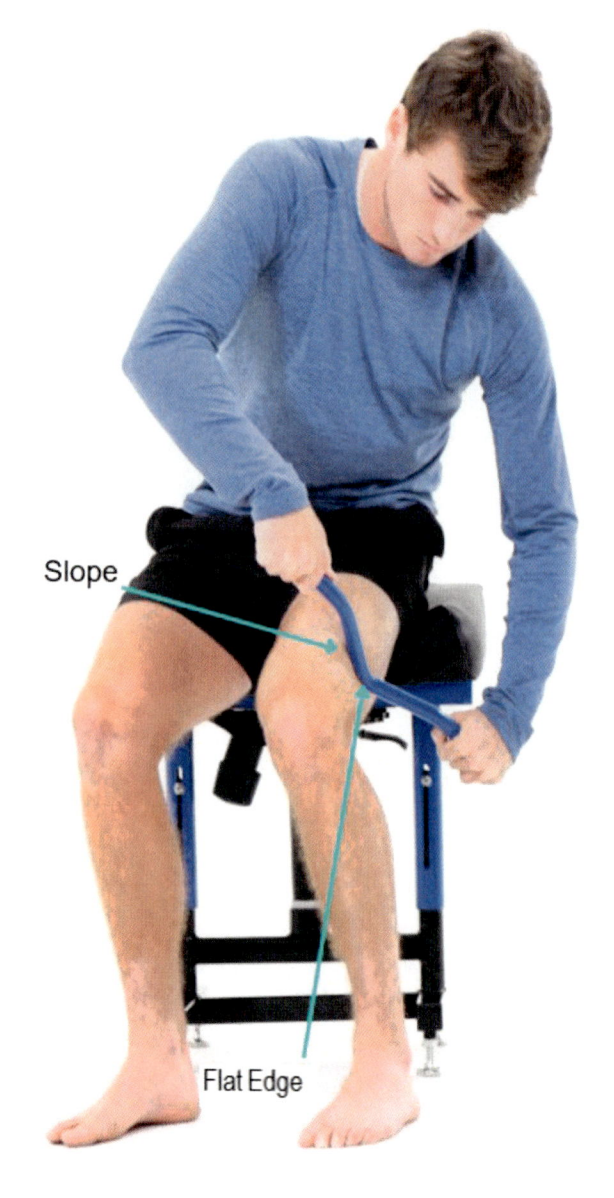

IT Band – Slope and Flat Edge

TIME:

15-30 seconds

BREATHING TECHNIQUE:

Breathe in for 3 seconds. As you exhale for 5 seconds, slide the TPRT up and down your IT Band with varying pressure.

TPRT MODULE 1 – SELF THERAPY

ADDUCTOR - INSIDE LEG - CURVE, POINT 1 & POINT 2

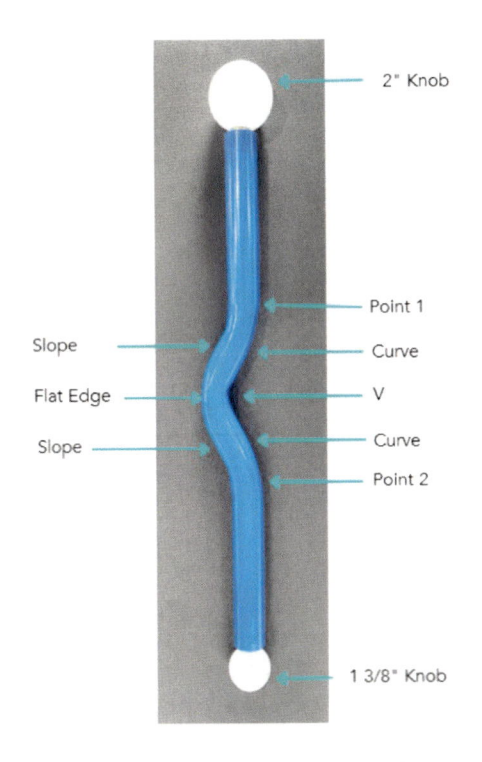

LUBRICATION: Lotion or oil

TPRT:
Use the Curves, V, Point 1, & 2

TECHNIQUE MOTION:
Use the Curve and the V to slide the TPRT up and down your adductors. Your bottom outside hand holds the tool stable while the top inside hand rocks the stick back and forth. This will allow you to use the Curves and the Points for more leverage.

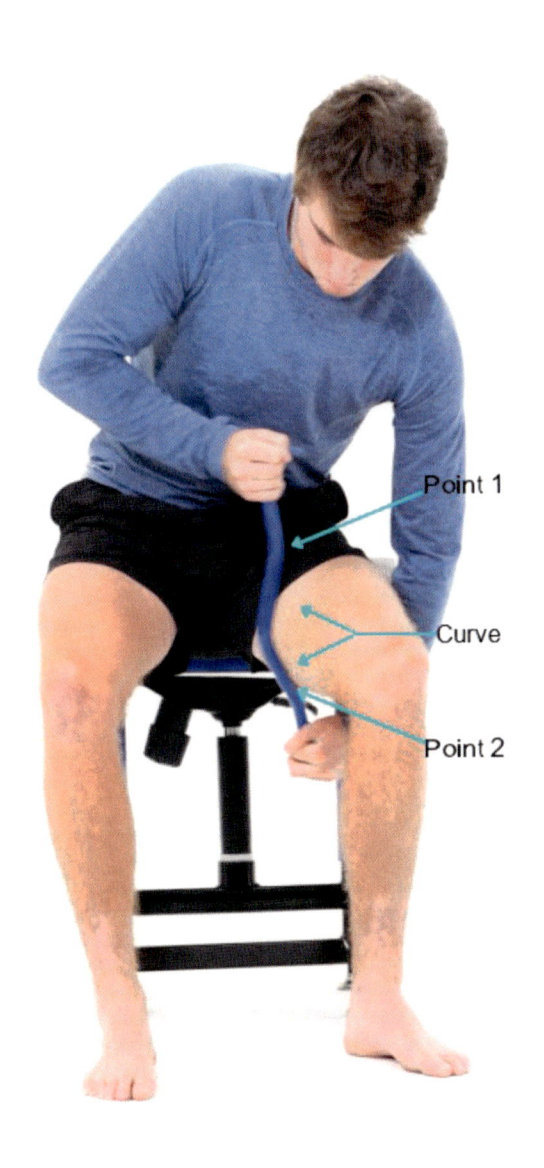

Adductor – Inside leg - Curve, Point 1, & 2

TIME:
15-30 seconds

BREATHING TECHNIQUE:
Breathe in for 3 seconds and slide the TPRT as you exhale for 5 seconds. Repeat four times.

TPRT MODULE 1 – SELF THERAPY

FRONT CALF - CURVE & POINT

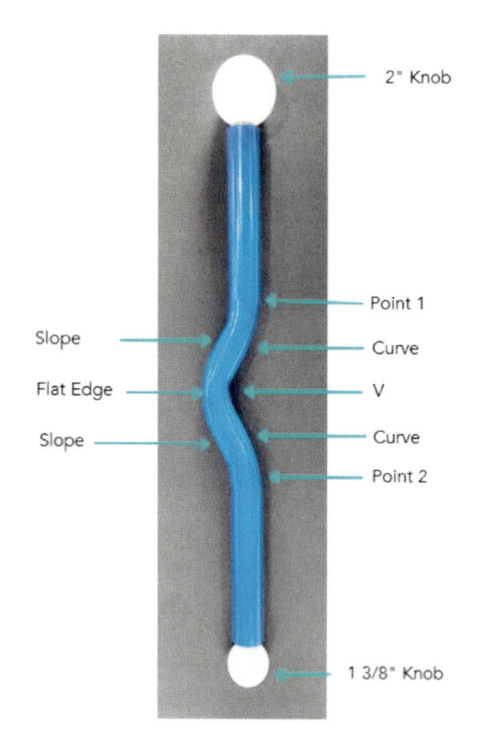

LUBRICATION: Lotion or oil

TPRT:

Use the Curve & Point 1

TECHNIQUE MOTION:

Use the Curve and Point 1 to **slide** the TPRT up and down your anterior calf muscles. Change angles and pressure by raising up the left hand and lowering the right and vice versa. This will allow you to use the Curves and the Points for more leverage.

TIME:

15-30 seconds

BREATHING TECHNIQUE:

Breathe in for 3 seconds. As you exhale for 5 seconds, slide the TPRT up and down your anterior calf with varying pressure.

Front Calf – Curve & Point 1

TPRT MODULE 1 – SELF THERAPY

FRONT CALF – PIN & ROCK - CURVE & POINT 1 OR 2

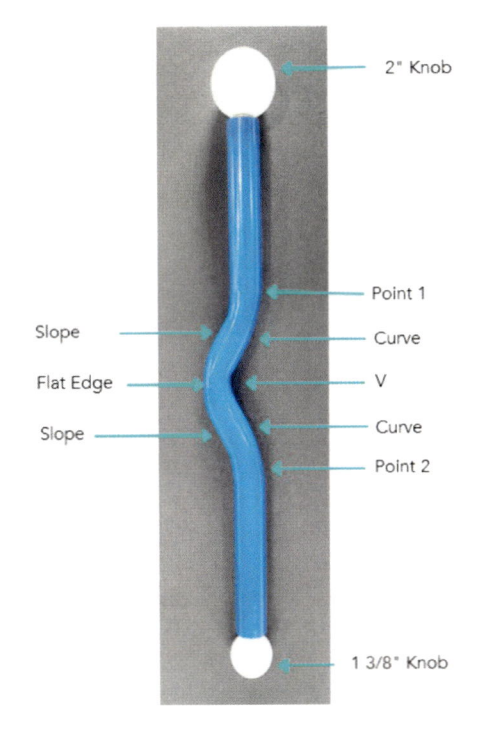

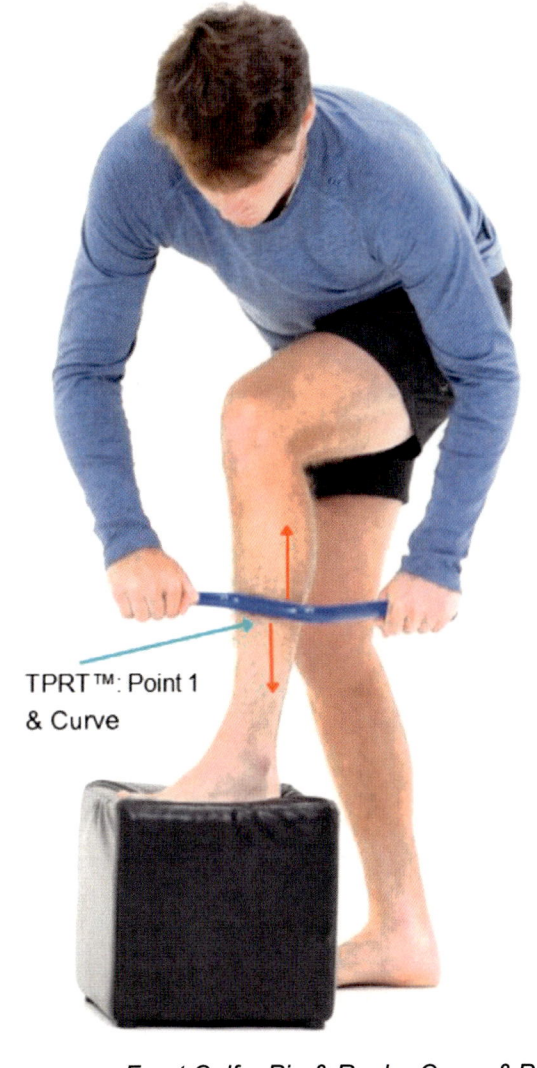

Front Calf – Pin & Rock – Curve & Point 1 or 2

LUBRICATION: none

TPRT:
Use the Curve & Point 1 or 2

TECHNIQUE MOTION:
Use the Curve and Point 1 or 2 to **Pin and Rock** the tissue. Use Point 1 to move the skin side to side, up and down, or move in small circles. Pick up the TPRT and move it to another portion of the front calf muscle to **pin and rock**. No lotion or oil is used in this technique. Change angles and pressure by raising up the left hand and lowering the right and vice versa. This will allow you to use the Curves and the Points for more leverage.

TIME:
15-30 seconds

BREATHING TECHNIQUE:
Breathe in for 3 seconds. As you exhale for 5 seconds, Pin and Rock the TPRT up and down your anterior calf with varying pressure.

TPRT MODULE 1 – SELF THERAPY

QUAD – PIN & ROCK - POINT 1 & CURVE

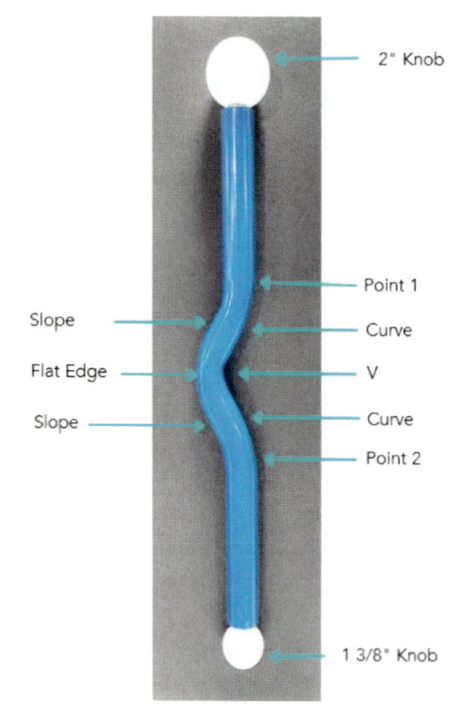

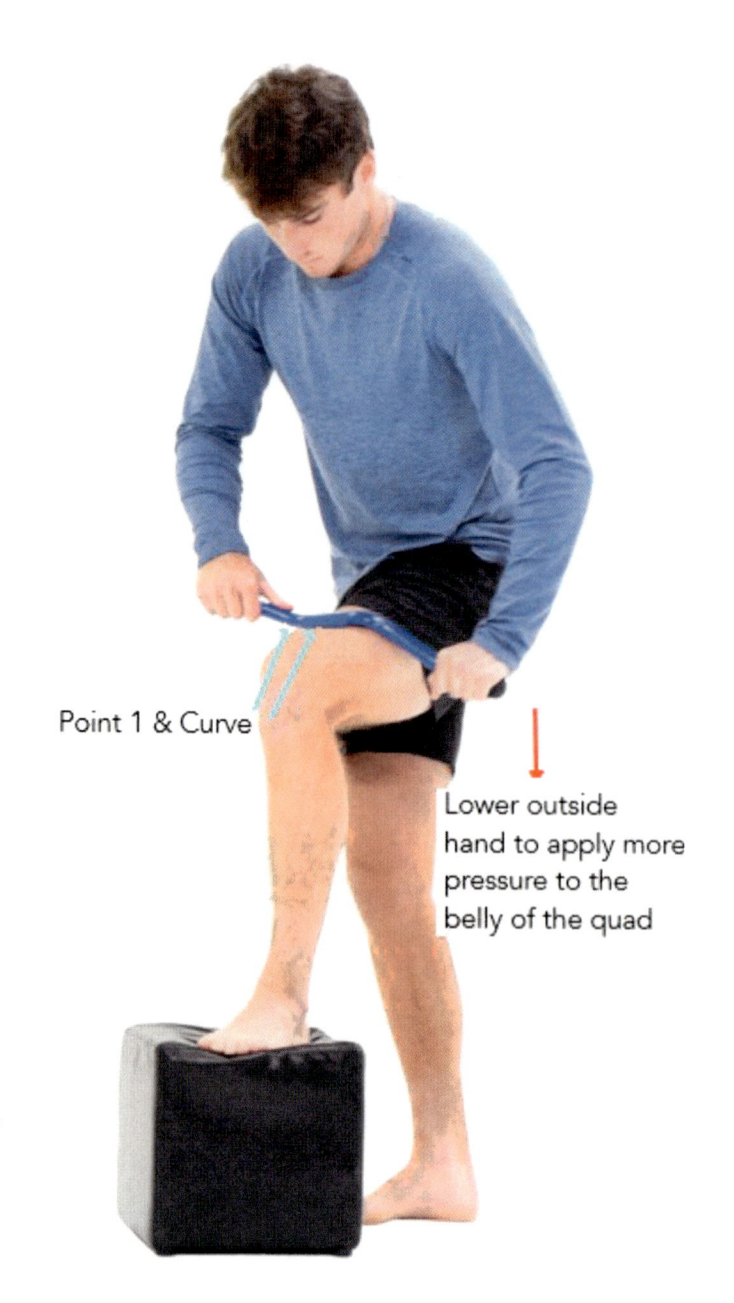

Labels on TPRT tool: 2" Knob, Slope, Flat Edge, Slope, Point 1, Curve, V, Curve, Point 2, 1 3/8" Knob

Point 1 & Curve

Lower outside hand to apply more pressure to the belly of the quad

LUBRICATION: None

TPRT:
Use the Curve & Point 1

TECHNIQUE MOTION:
Use the Curve and Point 1 to **Pin and Rock** the TPRT up and down your quad muscle just above the patella. *Change angles* and *pressure by raising up the left hand and lowering the right and vice versa.*

TIME:
15-30 seconds

Quad – Pin & Rock – Curve & Point 1

BREATHING TECHNIQUE:
Breathe in for 3 seconds. As you exhale for 5 seconds, **Pin and Rock** the TPRT up and down your quad muscle, moving tissue with varying pressure.

TPRT MODULE 1 – SELF THERAPY

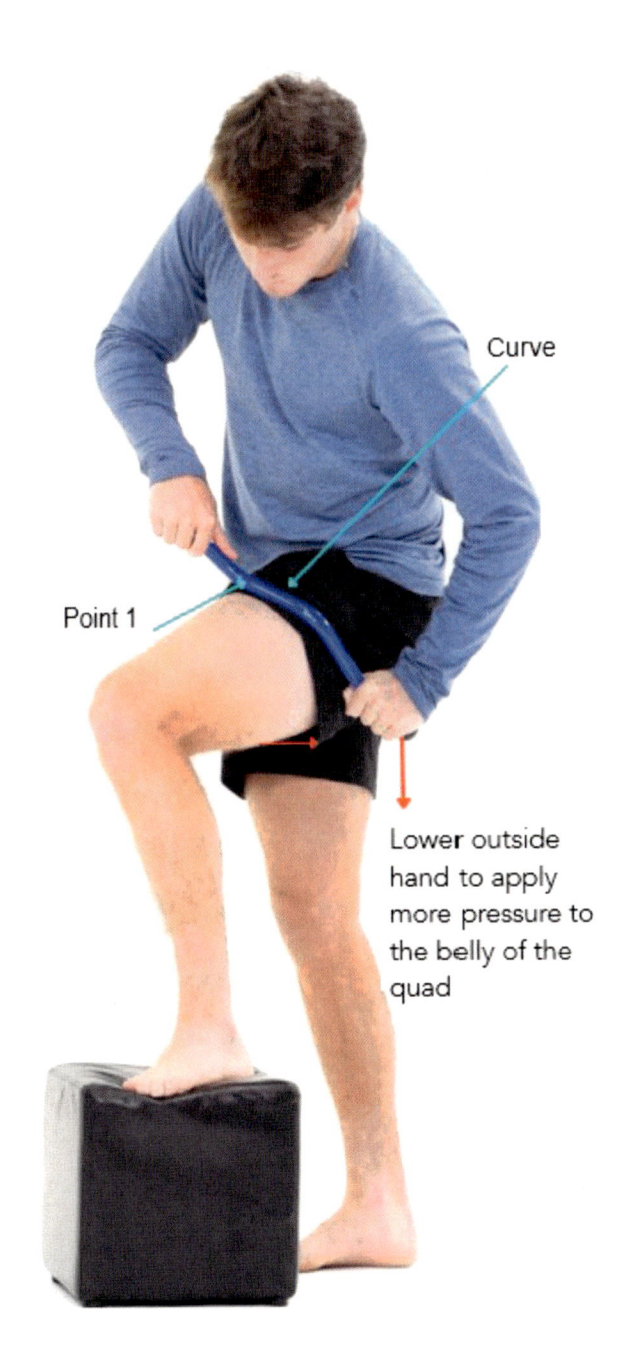

QUAD (INSIDE) PIN & RELEASE – CURVE & POINT 1

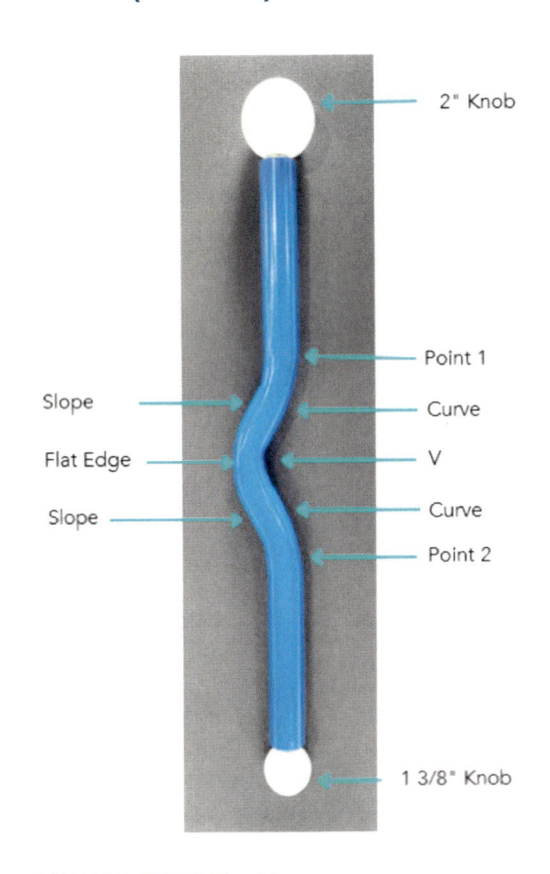

Labels on tool (left image): 2" Knob, Point 1, Slope, Curve, Flat Edge, V, Slope, Curve, Point 2, 1 3/8" Knob

Labels on demonstration (right image): Curve, Point 1, Lower outside hand to apply more pressure to the belly of the quad

LUBRICATION: None

TPRT:
Use the Curve & Point 1

TECHNIQUE MOTION:
<u>Pin and Release</u>. Pin the tissue; do not slide. Use Point 1 to apply more pressure to the right side to maneuver the skin up, down, and in circles.

TIME:
15-30 seconds

BREATHING TECHNIQUE:
Inhale for 3 seconds, then exhale for 5 seconds as you release the tissues.

Quad inside Pin & Release – Curve & Point 1

31

TPRT MODULE 1 – SELF THERAPY

QUAD (OUTSIDE) - INSIDE POINT 1

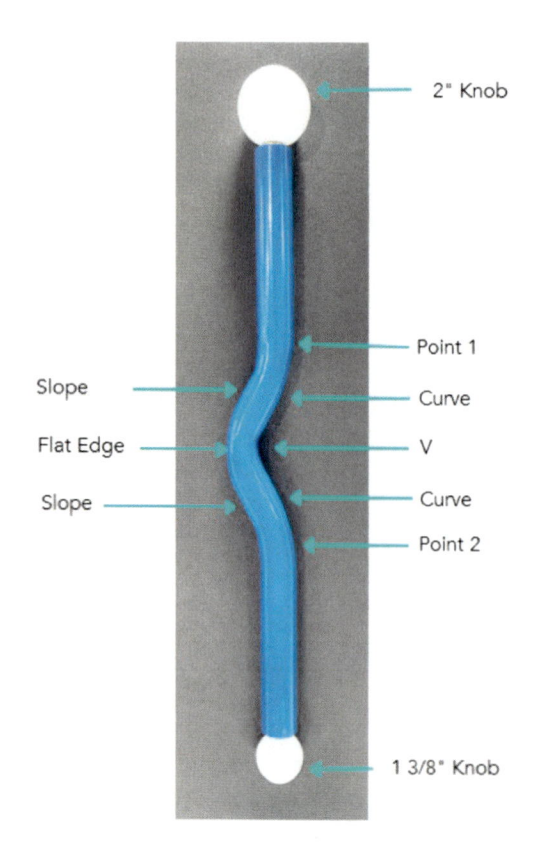

LUBRICATION: Lotion or Oil

TPRT:

Use the Curve & Point 1

TECHNIQUE MOTION:

Apply lotion to the tool and use the Point 1 angle to massage the outside of the leg.

TIME:

15-30 seconds

BREATHING TECHNIQUE:

Inhale for 3 seconds, then exhale for 5 seconds as you release the tissues.

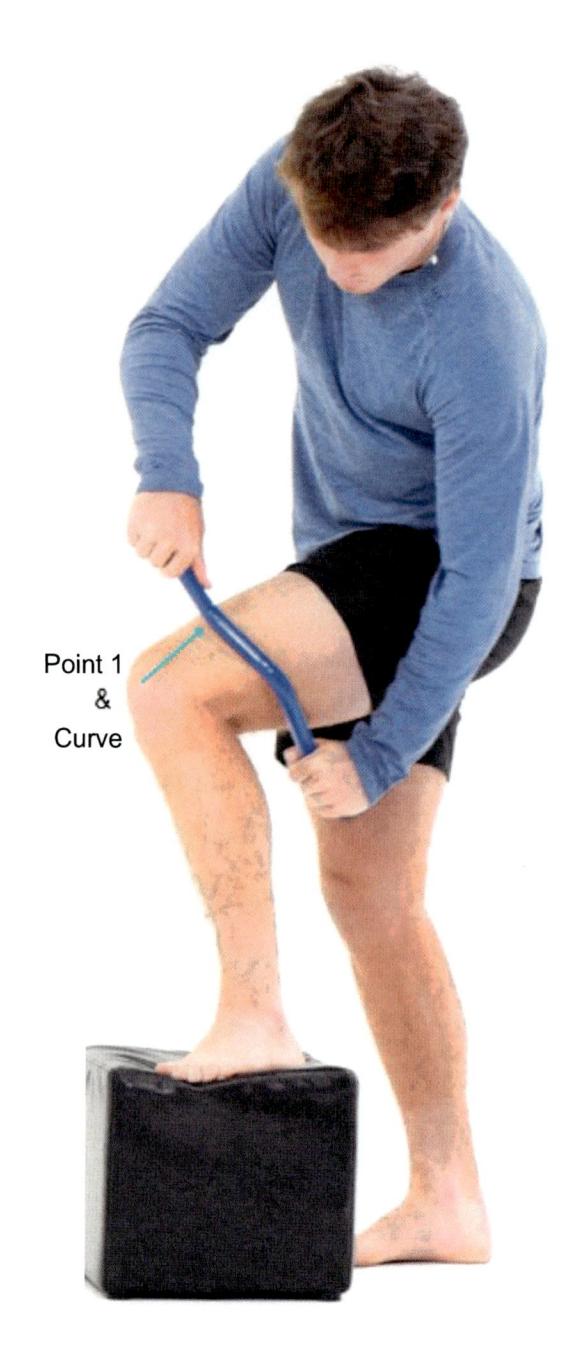

Quad (outside) - Point 1 & Curve

32

MEDIAL (INSIDE QUAD) – PIN & ROCK - POINT 2

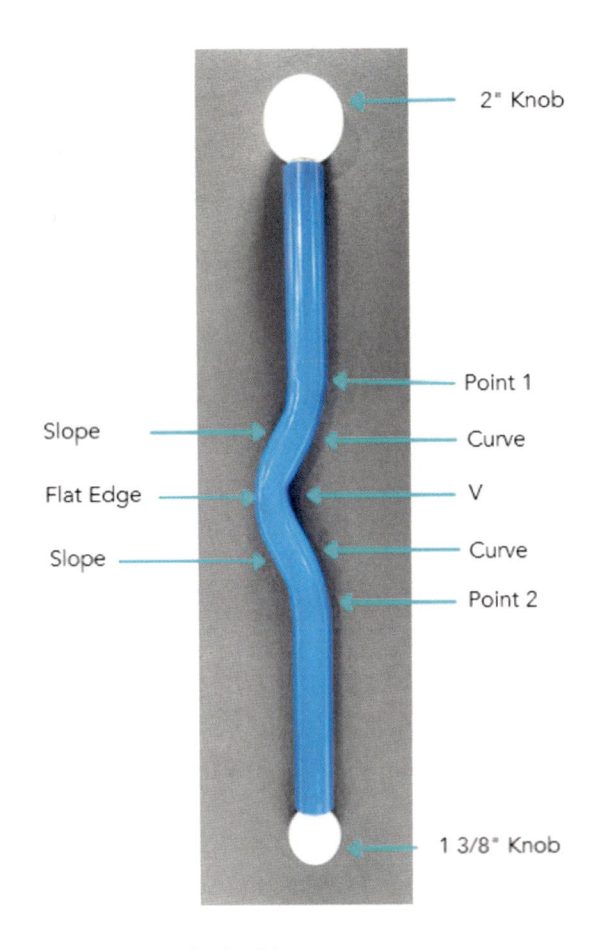

LUBRICATION: None

TPRT:

Use Point 2

TECHNIQUE MOTION:

Pin & Rock. Use Curve and Point 2 angle to rock the tool on the inside quad, e.g. (See-Saw Motion) 5 to 8 reps.

TIME:

15-30 seconds

BREATHING TECHNIQUE:

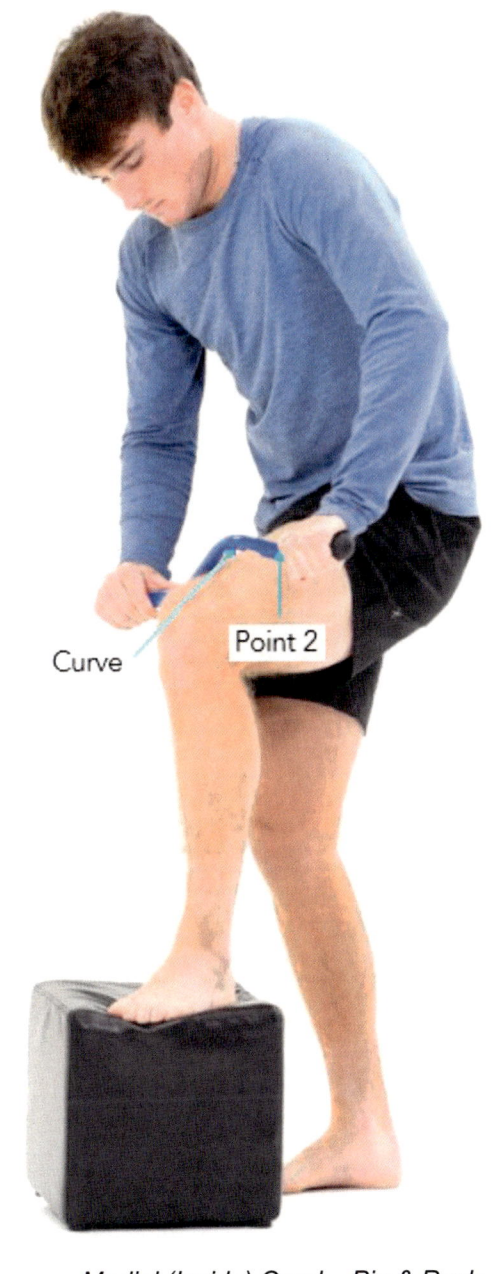

Inhale for 3 seconds, then exhale for 5 seconds as you release the tissues.

Medial (Inside) Quad – Pin & Rock – Point 2

TPRT MODULE 1 – SELF THERAPY

BACK (POSTERIOR) CALF - CURVES

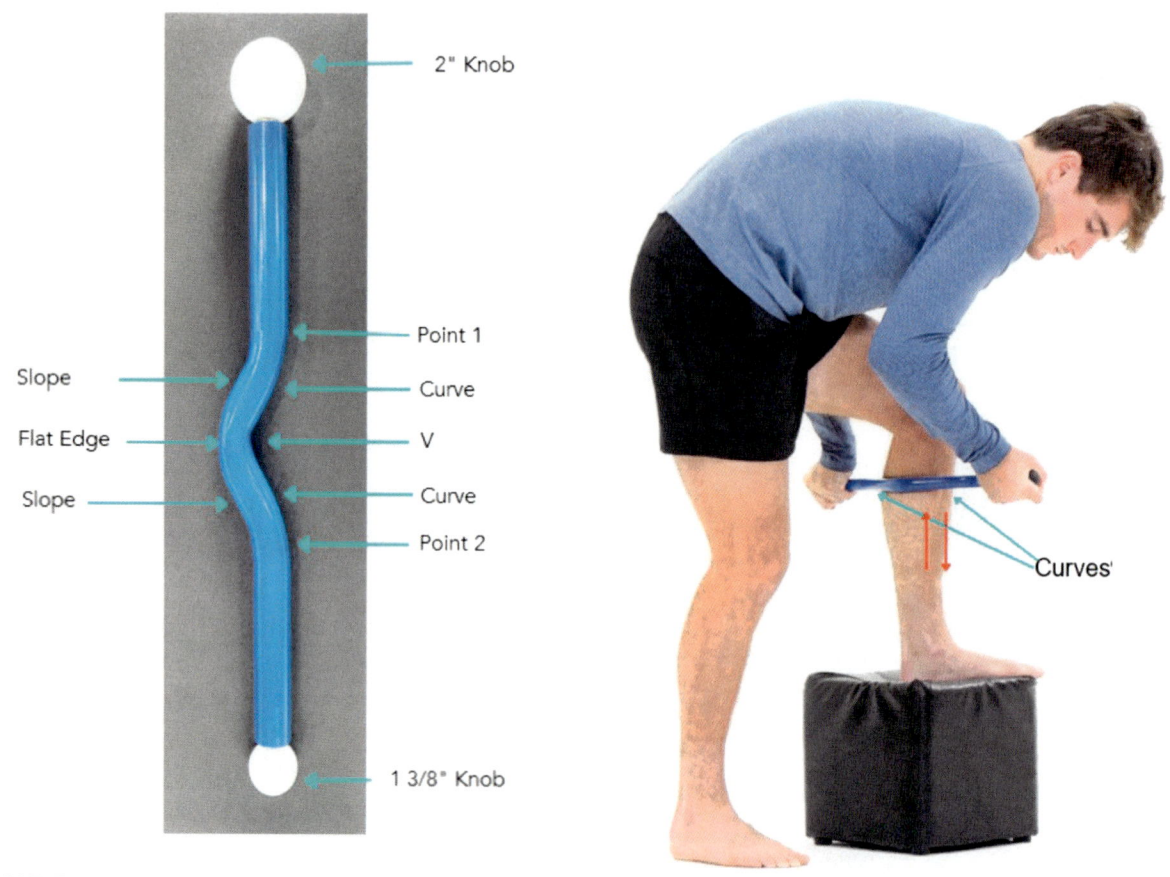

Back Calf - Curves

LUBRICATION: Lotion or Oil

TPRT:
Use Curves

TECHNIQUE MOTION:
Apply lotion and <u>slide</u> the Curve up and down. Apply equal pressure to each side of the tool.

TIME:
15-30 seconds

BREATHING TECHNIQUE:
Inhale for 3 seconds, then exhale for 5 seconds as you release the tissues.

TPRT MODULE 1 – SELF THERAPY

LOW BACK OVER SHIRT– POINT 1 & 2

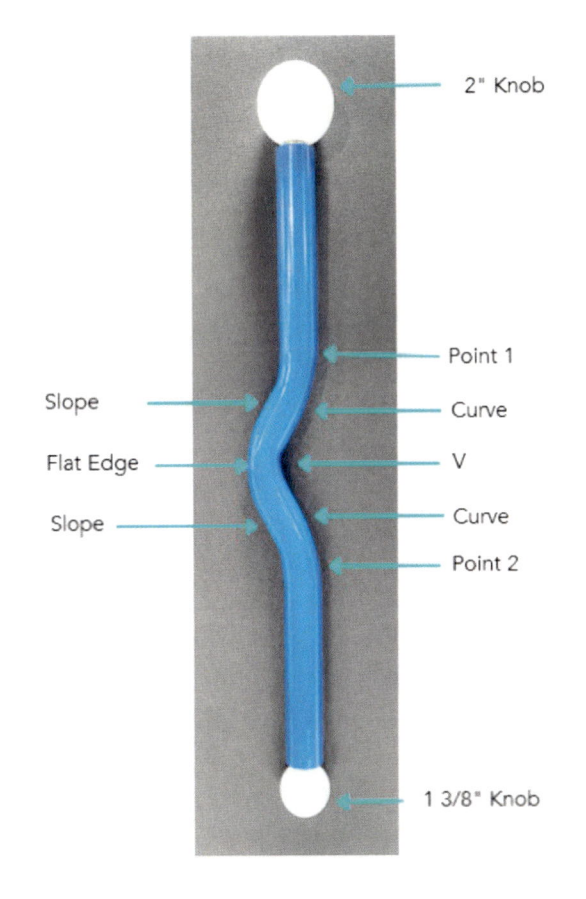

LUBRICATION: None

TPRT:
Use Curves, Point 1 & 2

TECHNIQUE MOTION:
Slide the TPRT up and down over a shirt.

TIME:
15-30 seconds

BREATHING TECHNIQUE:
Inhale for 3 seconds, then exhale for 5 seconds as you release the tissues.

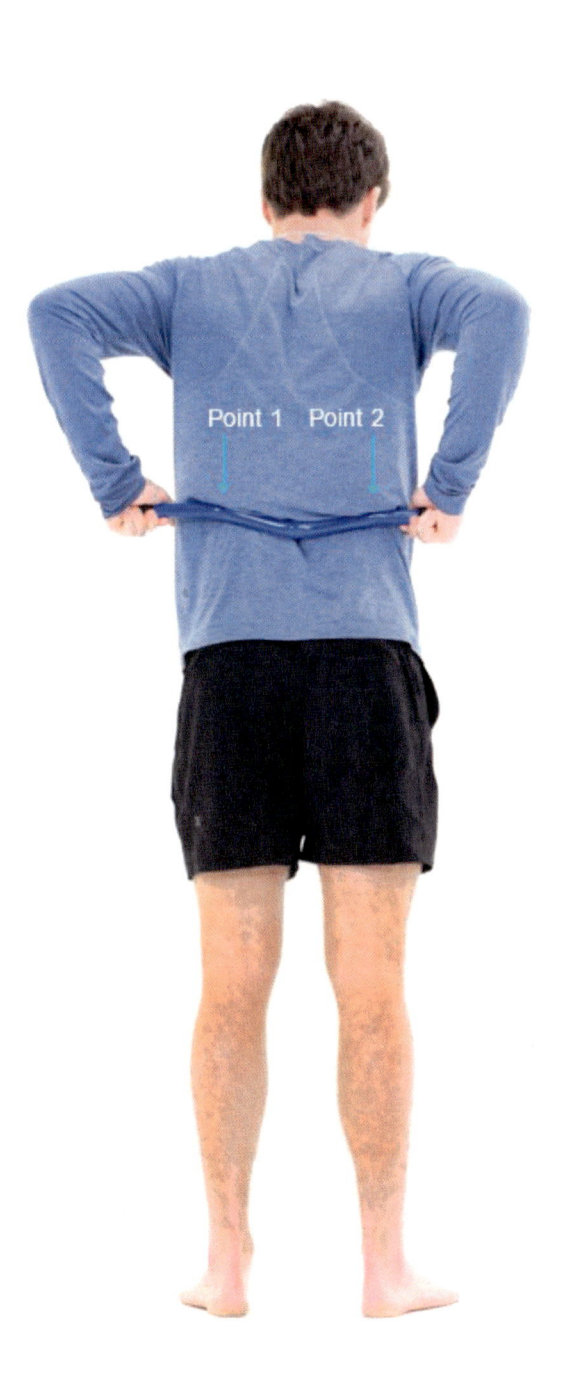

Low back – Curves, Point 1 & 2

35

TPRT MODULE 1 – SELF THERAPY

ABS – FLAT EDGE OVER SHIRT

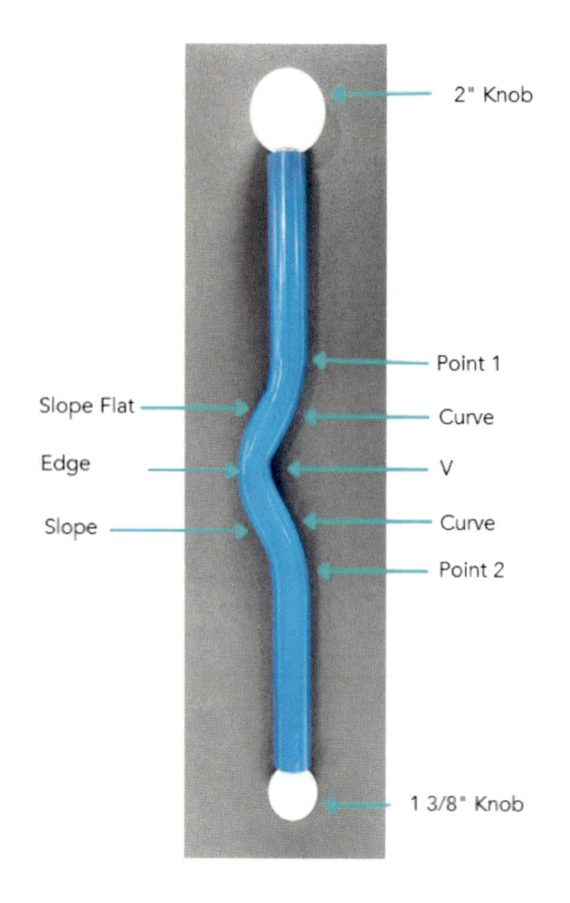

(Tool diagram labeled: 2" Knob, Point 1, Slope Flat, Curve, Edge, V, Slope, Curve, Point 2, 1 3/8" Knob)

LUBRICATION: None

TPRT:
Use Flat Edge

TECHNIQUE MOTION:
<u>Slide</u> up and down. Slide the Flat Edge up and find your ribs. Work below your ribs on your abs.

TIME:
15-30 seconds

BREATHING TECHNIQUE:
Inhale for 3 seconds, then exhale for 5 seconds a you release the tissues.

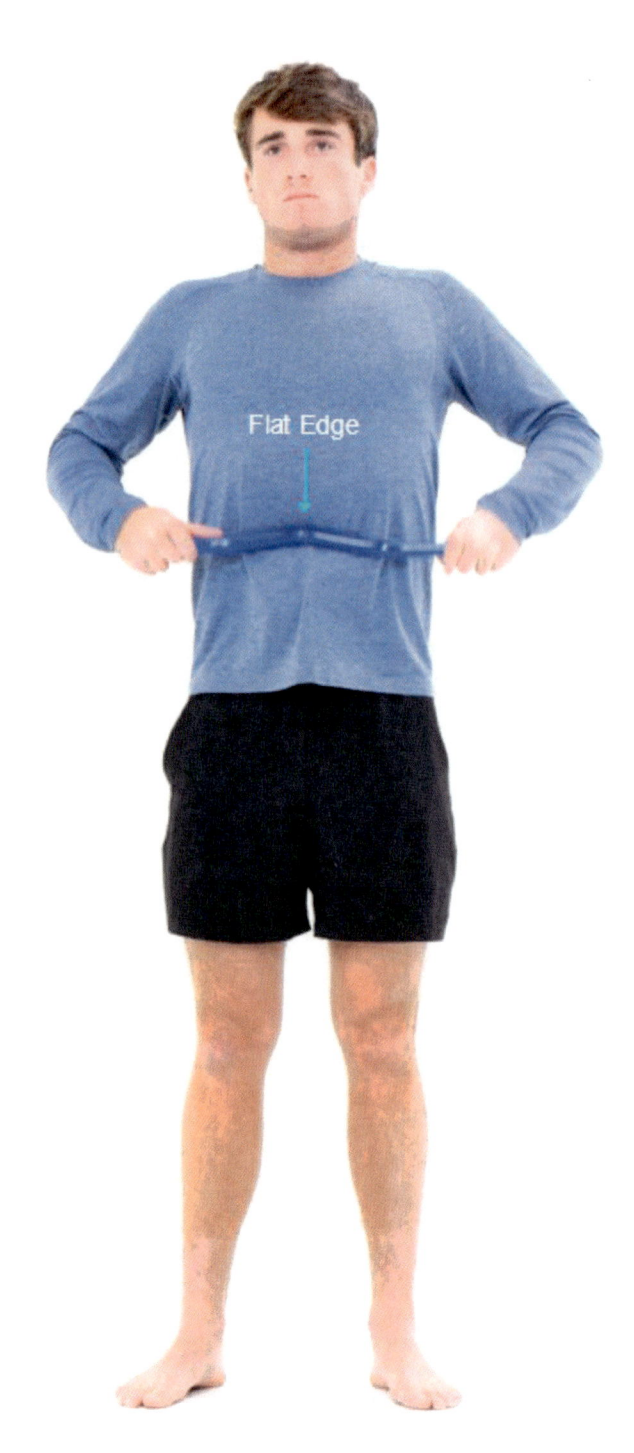

Abs Flat Edge over shirt

OUTSIDE ABS – FLAT EDGE OVER SHIRT

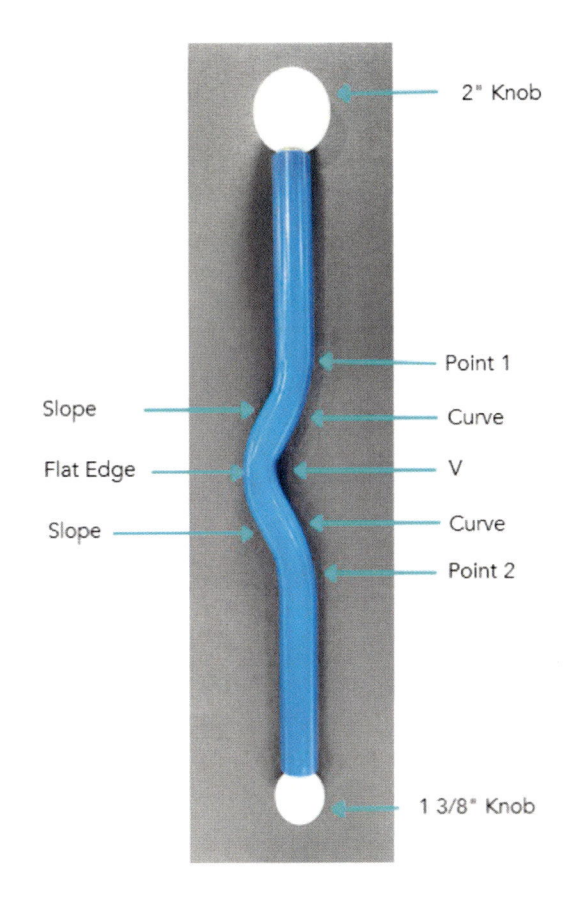

LUBRICATION: None

TPRT:
Use Flat Edge.

TECHNIQUE MOTION:
Slide up and down. Slide the Flat Edge up and down on the muscles. Repeat on the other side.

TIME:
15-30 seconds

BREATHING TECHNIQUE:
Inhale for 3 seconds, then exhale for 5 seconds as you release the tissues.

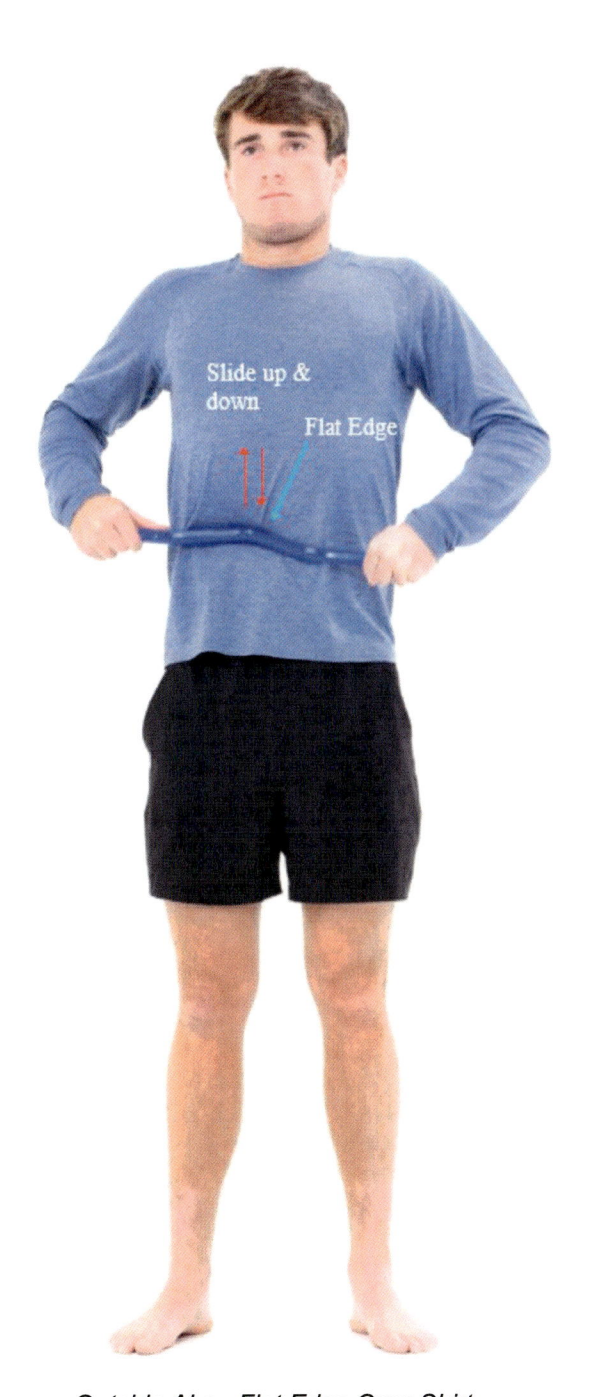

Outside Abs - Flat Edge Over Shirt

MEDIAL (INSIDE) FOREARM – SMALL KNOB

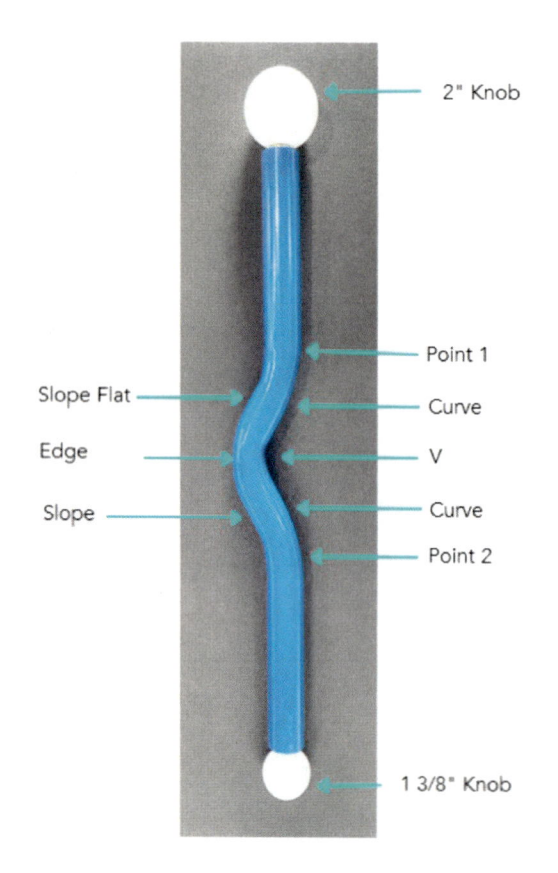

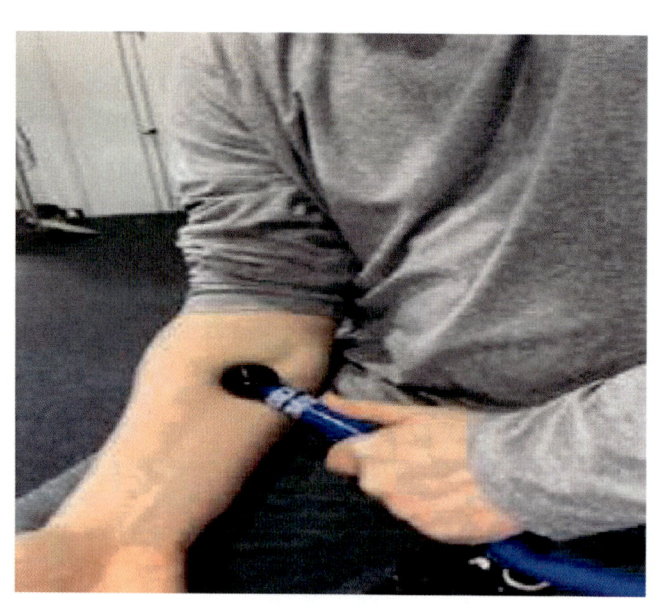

Medial (Inside) Right Forearm – Small Knob

LUBRICATION: None

TPRT:

Small Knob

TECHNIQUE MOTION:

Pin and move the muscle up and down. Use the 1 3/8" knob to pin and release muscles on your forearm.

Then repeat moving the knob to a different location. Either up towards your elbow or down towards your wrist. Apply Pressure on exhale.

TIME:

15-30 seconds

BREATHING TECHNIQUE:

Breathe in for 3 seconds. As you exhale for 5 seconds, Pin and move the TPRT up and down your medial (inside) forearm, moving tissues with varying pressure.

TRPT MODULE 2 – CLIENT THERAPY

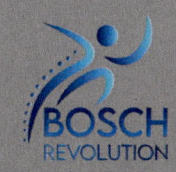

The Client Therapy module is designed for Massage Therapists, Physical Therapists, Athletic Trainers, and Movement Specialists. Here you will learn how to use the TPRT with your clients.

The TPRT is unique because the knobs are made of FDA-approved rubber nitrile, which provides a tactile connection on the skin that allows you to release trigger points and to move fascia. The Curves and Contours enable you to cover more surface area on the skin and apply leverage onto the muscles.

In this module, we will address the following:
- core
- hips
- lower back
- legs
- feet
- back
- shoulders
- arms
- forearms
- neck
- trunk

Important questions to ask your client or have on your intake form when working on them with the Trigger Point Release Tool™

- Do you have localized pain in your muscles?
- Is the pain worse when pressure is applied to the muscle?
- Do you experience referring pain, meaning that the pain radiates from the trigger point to another area of your body?
- Is the pain worse at certain times of the day or after specific activities?
- Do you have a reduced range of motion in the affected muscle? Do you feel fatigued in specific muscles?
- Do your muscles feel tight or knotted?

AB RELEASE (SUPINE 1) – SLOPE

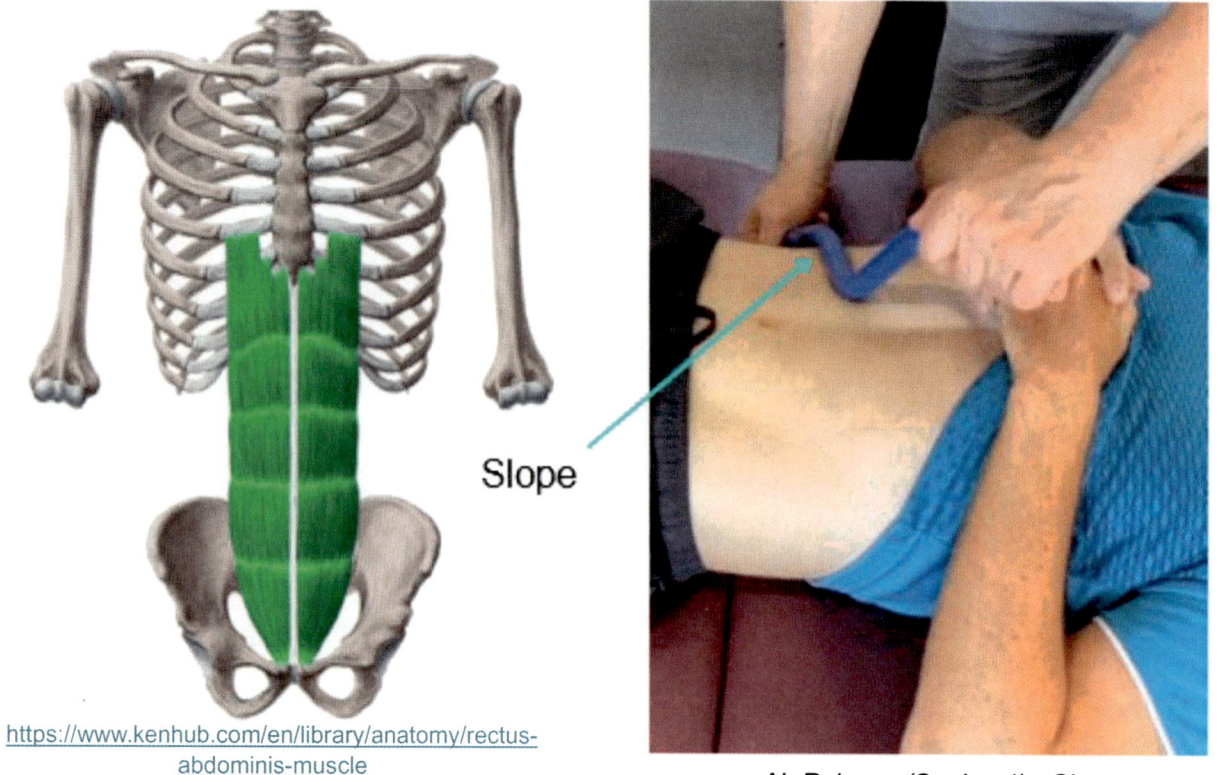

Ab Release (Supine 1) - Slope

LUBRICATION: Lotion or Oil

TPRT:

Slope

TECHNIQUE MOTION:

The therapist stands above the hips.

Apply oil or lotion to the skin first - Use the Slope to slide from just below the right rib and move down past the belly button using the Slope.

Remember to ensure your client has not just eaten, as this could be uncomfortable for them.

AB RELEASE (SUPINE 2) – SLOPE

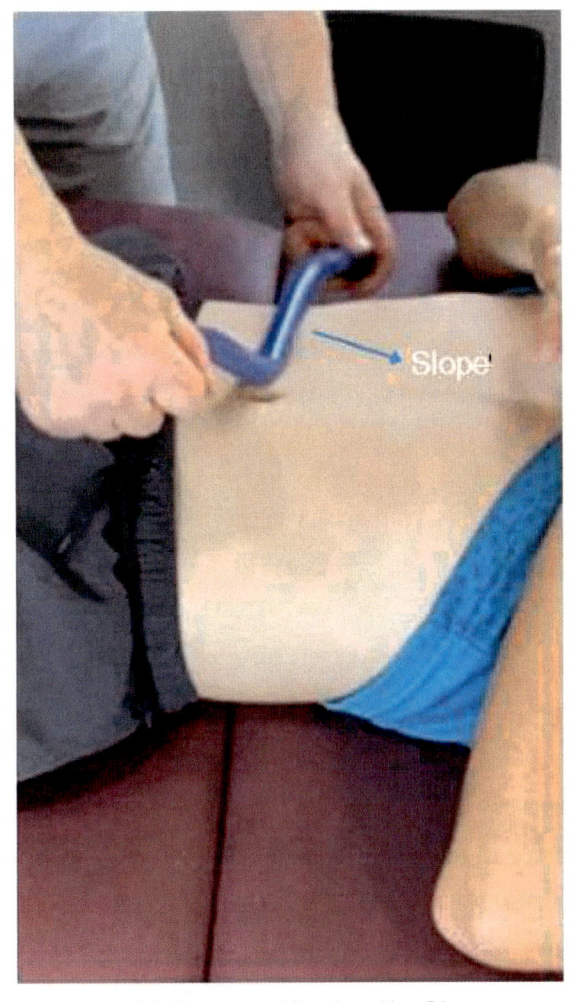

Ab Release (Supine 2) - Slope

LUBRICATION: Lotion or Oil

TPRT:

Slope

TECHNIQUE MOTION:

The therapist stands below the hips.

First, apply oil or lotion to the skin. Then, use the Slope to <u>slide</u> from just below the belly button up to the right rib.

Remember to ensure your client has not just eaten, as this could be uncomfortable for them.

TPRT MODULE 2 – CLIENT THERAPY

ILIACUS RELEASE – SMALL KNOB

Trigger points in the iliacus can refer sensations to in the groin, hip, lower back, the sacroiliac joint, and down the leg. A tight iliacus can lead to a functional leg length difference and promote pelvic torsion.

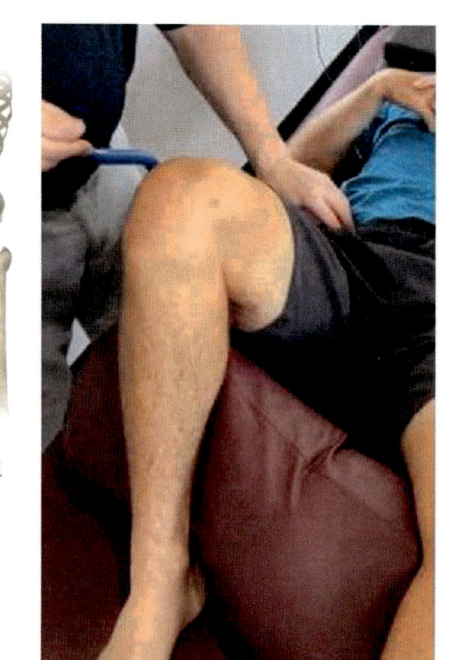

LUBRICATION: None

TPRT:

Small Knob

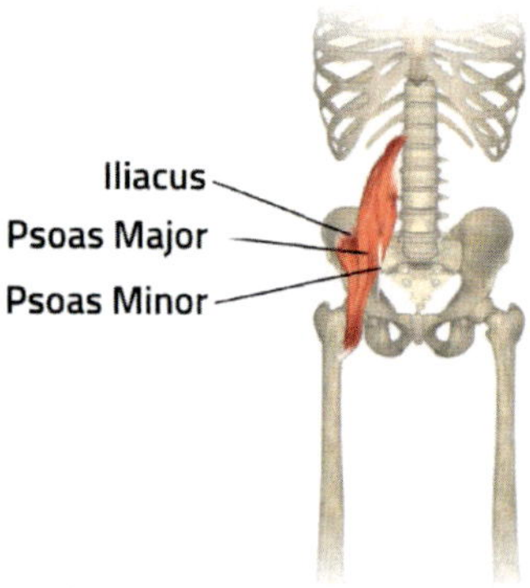

TECHNIQUE MOTION:

The therapist stands at hip level.

Find the ASIS with your fingers. Find the bone and slide it into the iliac fossa. Place the small knob just inside the iliac fossa. Be sure that you are not on the inguinal ligament.

https://3dmusclelab.com/wp-content/uploads/2019/01/iliacus-psoas.jpg

Place the small knob on the ASIS.

Have the client inhale. On the exhale, gently apply pressure.

Inguinal Ligament: A set of two bands deep in the groin connects the oblique muscles of the abdomen to the pelvis. They support soft tissue in the groin area and anchor the abdomen and pelvis.

https://www.painreliefvermont.com/iliacus-dysfunction

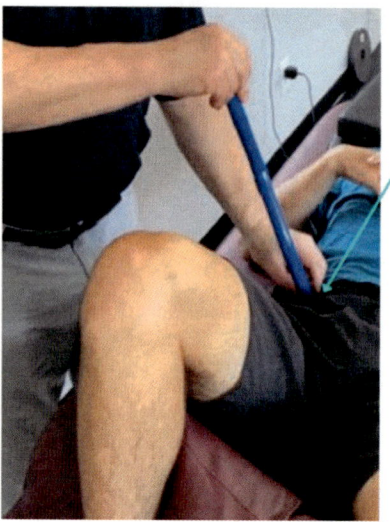

Iliacus Release – Small Knob

TPRT MODULE 2 – CLIENT THERAPY

PSOAS DISTAL ATTACHMENT (SIDE LYING) – SMALL KNOB

LUBRICATION: None

TPRT:

Small Knob

TECHNIQUE MOTION:

Find the posterior portion of the femur with your fingers. Then place the small knob and move towards the midline. The common tendon attaches to the lesser Trochanter of the femur. The muscles, during contraction of the fibers, lead to flexion and external rotation of the hip and bends the lumbar vertebral column.

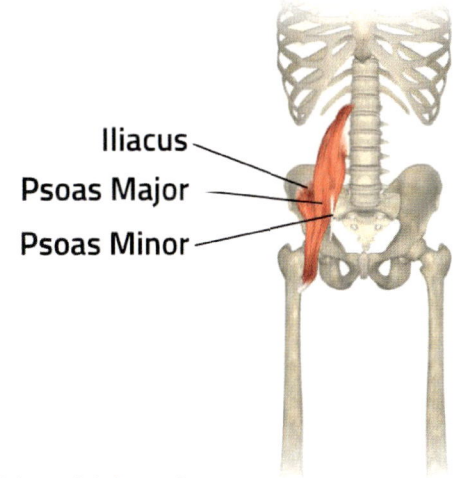

https://3dmusclelab.com/wp-content/uploads/2019/01/iliacus-psoas.jpg

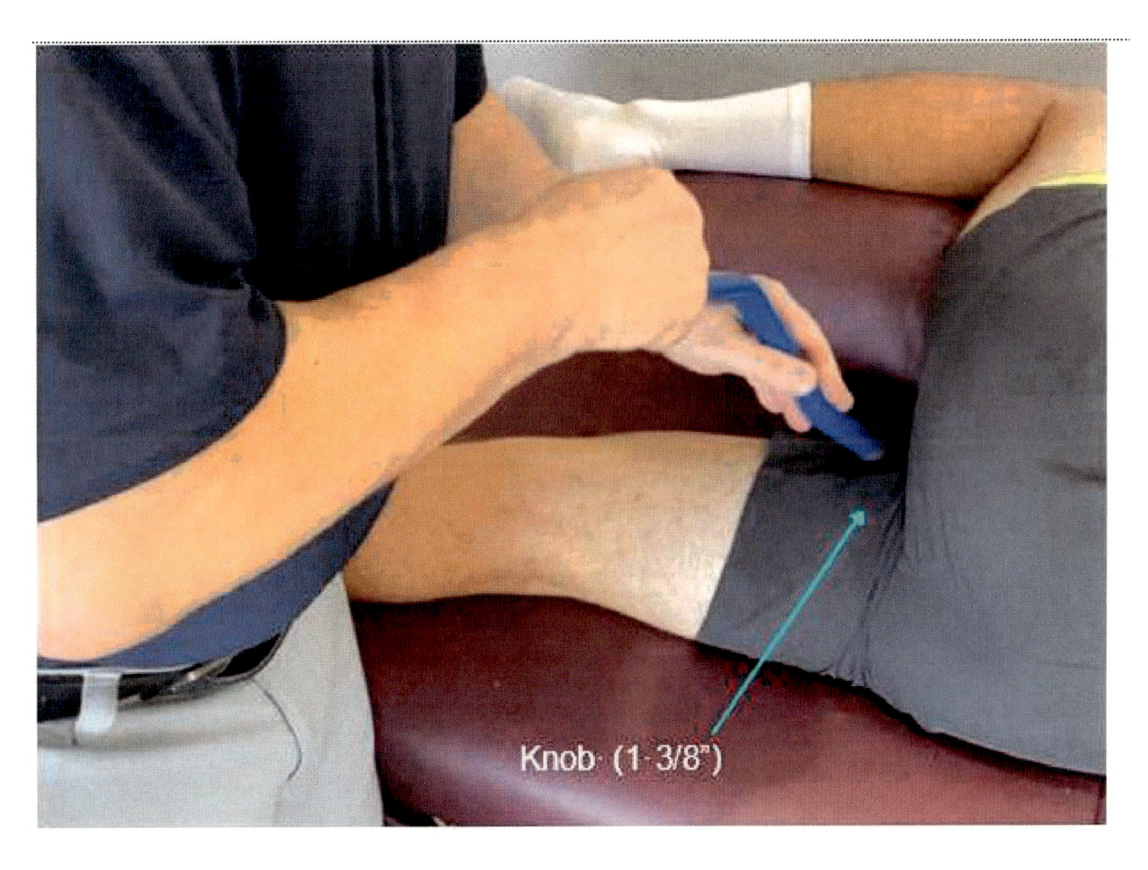

Psoas Distal Attachment – Small Knob

AB RELEASE (STANDING): RECTUS ABDOMINUS - SLOPES

EDUCATION:

The rectus abdominus is a large muscle located on either side of the abdomen, which can give the appearance of a six-pack.

The muscle extends from an area of the pelvis (pubis symphysis) to the lower ribs.

The rectus abdominus helps to maintain an upright posture and flex (bend) the lumbar spine (lower back).

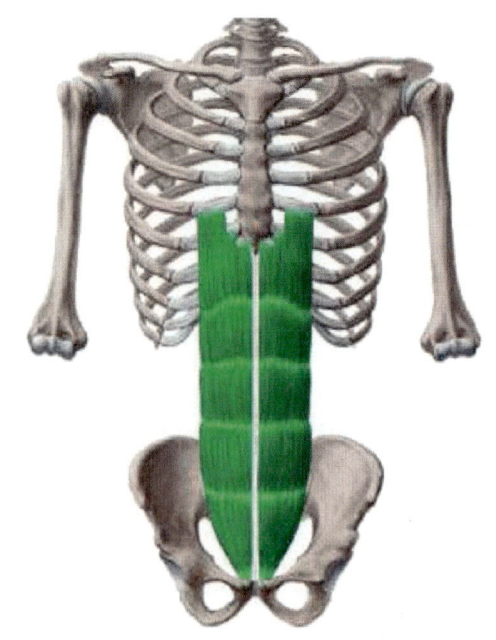

https://www.kenhub.com/en/library/anatomy/rectus-abdominis-muscle

LUBRICATION: Oil or Lotion

TPRT:

Slopes

TECHNIQUE MOTION:

Apply lotion or oil to the rectus abdominus muscle.

In a standing position, place the TPRT just below the ribs. Use the Slopes to slide down the rectus abdomens (abs). You can go to the pubic bone or stop just below the belly button.

You may want to release this in a supine position with the legs bent to work lower abs.

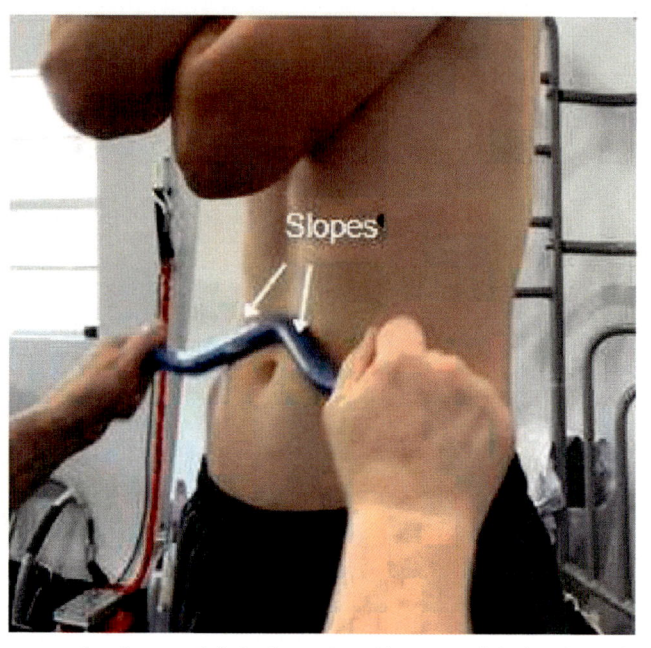

www.physio.co.uk/what-we-treat/surgery/abdominals/rectus-abdominis-repair.php

TPRT™ MODULE 3 – CLIENT THERAPY

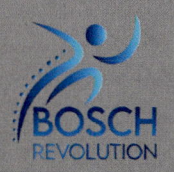

FOREARM

EDUCATION:

The anterior or volar compartment of the forearm contains eight muscles: five belong to the superficial group (pronator teres, flexor carpi radialis, palmaris longus, flexor digitorum superficialis, and flexor carpi ulnaris), and three to the deep group (flexor digitorum profundus, flexor pollicis longus, and pronator quadratus).

The flexor digitorum profundus (FDP) muscle makes up the third layer of the anterior compartment of the forearm along with the flexor pollicis longus muscle. It passes through the carpal tunnel and is one of the extrinsic muscles of the hand.

Origin:
- Medial olecranon, upper three-quarters of the anterior and medial surface of ulna, adjacent interosseous membrane.
- Shares aponeurotic attachment to the posterior border of the ulna with flexor & extensor carpi ulnaris.

Insertion: volar surface of distal phalanges of the second to fifth fingers.

Anterior

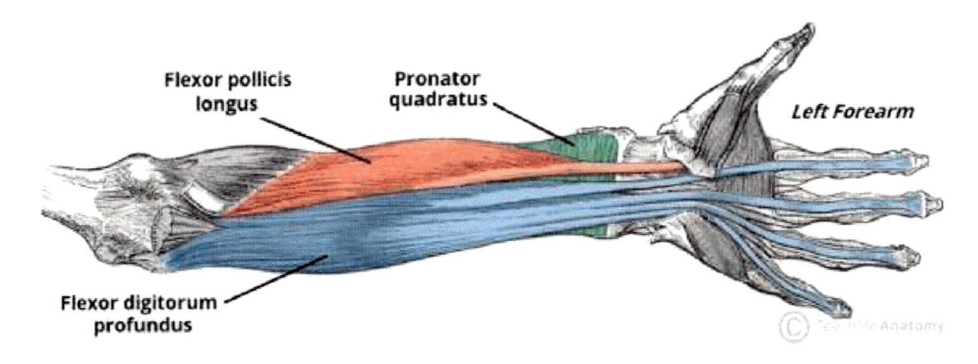

Left Forearm

https://teachmeanatomy.info/wp-content/uploads/Deep-Flexor-Muscles-of-the-Anterior-Forearm.png.webp

Forearm (Supine): Flexor Carpi Radialis, Palmaris Longus, Flexor Digitorum Superficialis

45

FOREARM – SLOPE

PART 1

LUBRICATION:
Oil or Lotion

TPRT:
Slope

TECHNIQUE MOTION:

Apply oil or lotion to the anterior forearm. Use the Slope of the TPRT to slide up the forearm. Have the client slowly make a fist and then open their hand as you slide up and down the forearm.

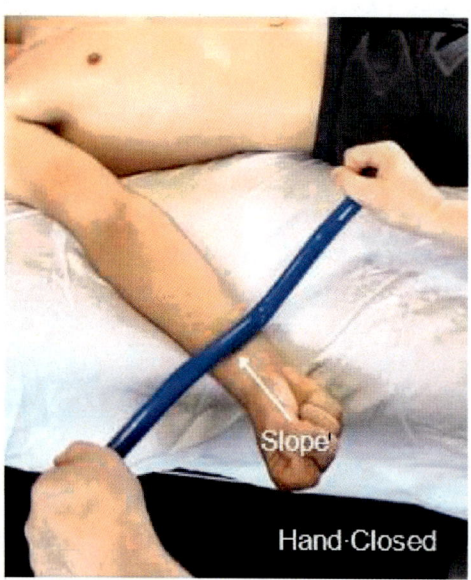

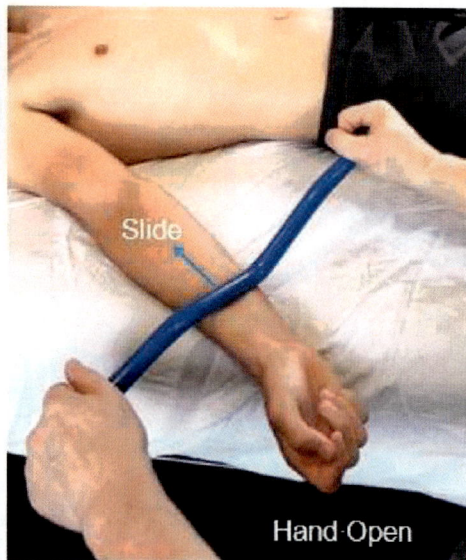

Forearm - Slope

PART 2

LUBRICATION: None

TPRT:
Slope

TECHNIQUE MOTION:

Place the Slope on the middle of the anterior forearm.

Have the client slowly make a fist and then close their hand as you Pin And Release their forearm muscles.

Repeat this 3 or 4 times, then move up or down. You may want to use your hands to palpate the forearm muscles and locate other trigger points to release.

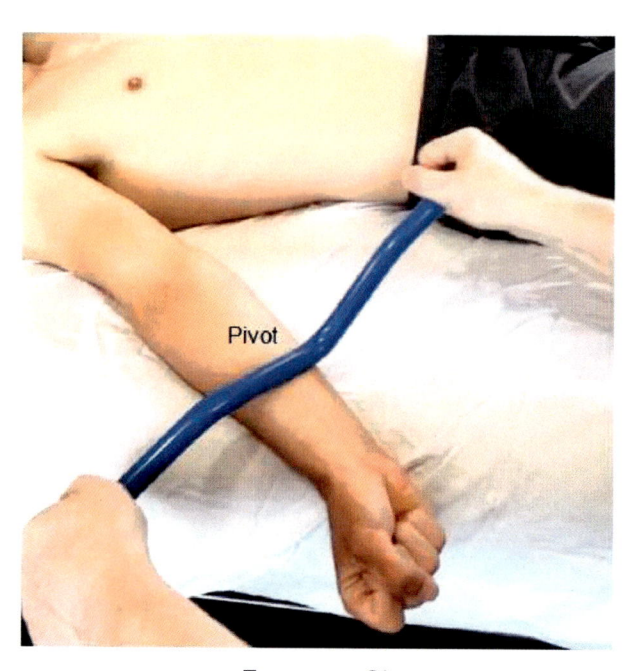

Forearm - Slope

ANTERIOR FOREARM (SIDE LYING)–CURVE, SLOPE, FLAT EDGE

LUBRICATION: Oil or Lotion

TPRT:

Curve, Slope, Flat Edge

TECHNIQUE MOTION:

Superficial: Release the Pronator Teres, Brachioradialis, Flexor Carpi Radialis, Palmaris Longus.

Deep: Flexor Digitorum Superficialis, Flexor Palmaris longus. Apply lotion and <u>slide</u> up and down using the Curve or the Slope.

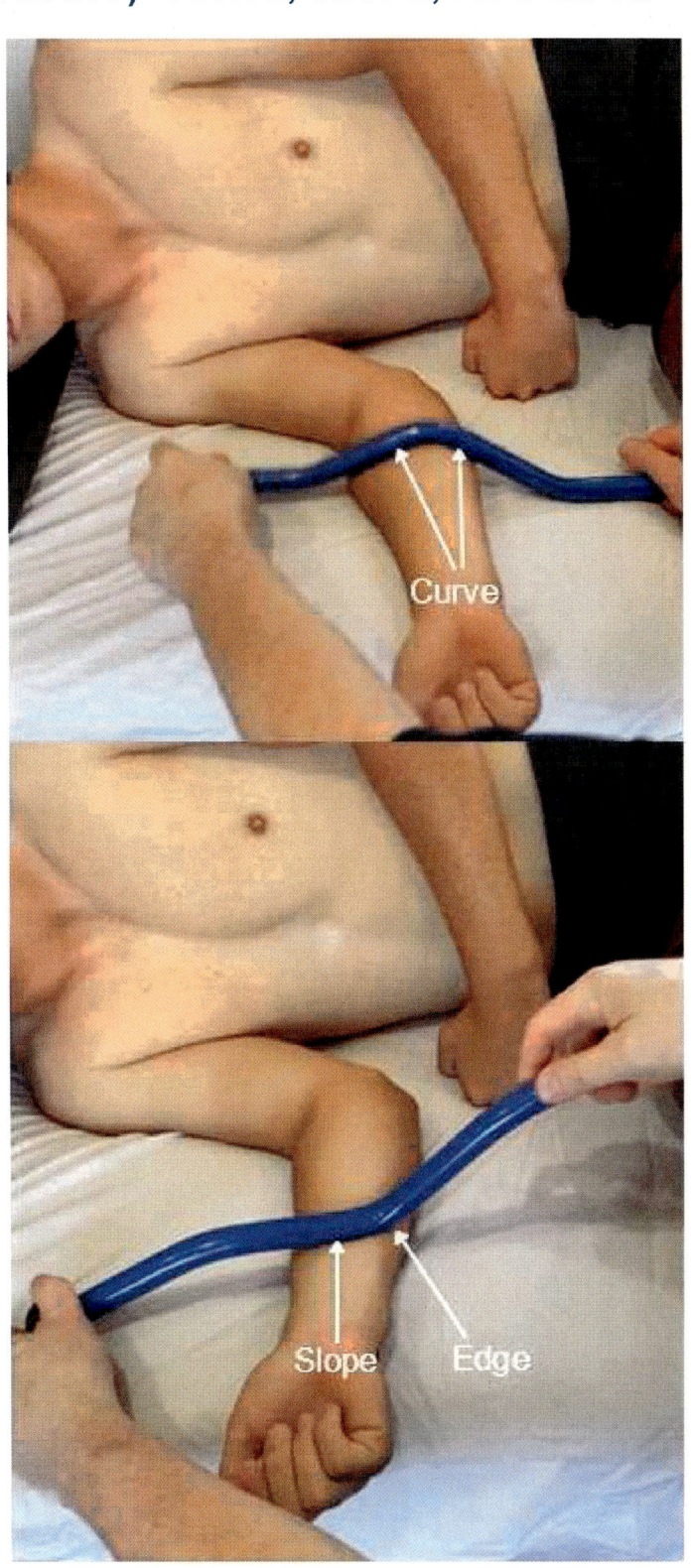

Anterior Forearm – Curve, Slope, Flat Edge

ANTERIOR FOREARM (SIDE LYING)–CURVE, SLOPE, FLAT EDGE

LUBRICATION: None

TPRT:
Small Knob

TECHNIQUE MOTION:
Supinate wrist. Use the knob just inside the most medial part of the ulna. Use the small knob to engage the skin and muscles of the Flexor Carpi Ulnaris, Flexor Digitorum Profundus, and Flexor Digitorum Superficialis.

When releasing muscles, breathe in for 3 seconds as you exhale to a five-count, applying pressure to the tissues.

Work medial to lateral. Place the small knob just inside of the ulna bone and release.

#1 Flexor Carpi Ulnaris, move in slightly to

#2 Palmaris Longus followed by

#3 Flexor Carpi Radialis and

#4 Pronator Teres

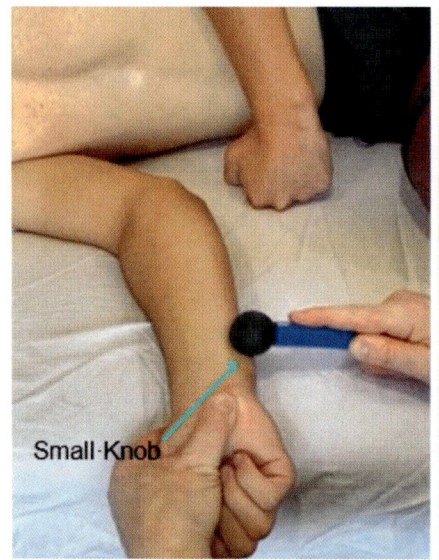

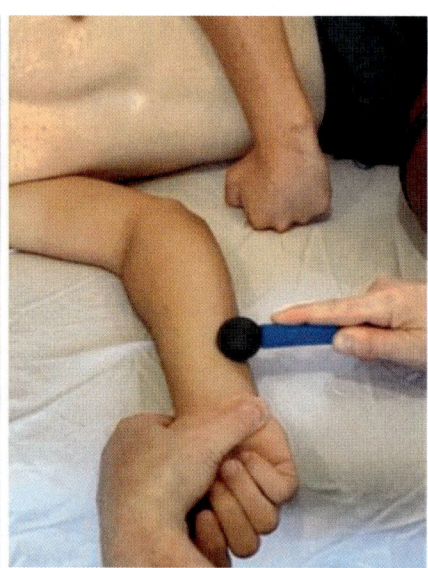

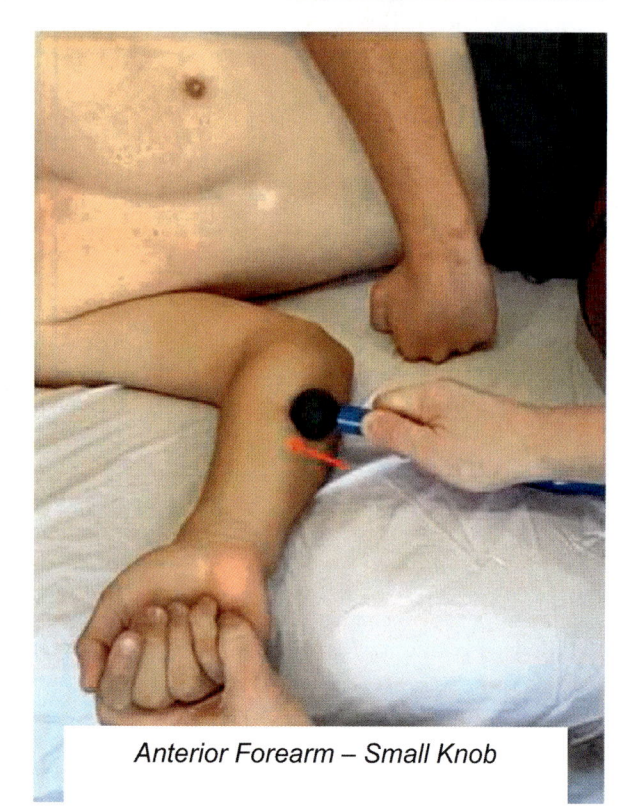

Anterior Forearm – Small Knob

ANTERIOR FOREARM (SUPINE) – CURVE

EDUCATION:

Superficial Layer of the Posterior Compartment

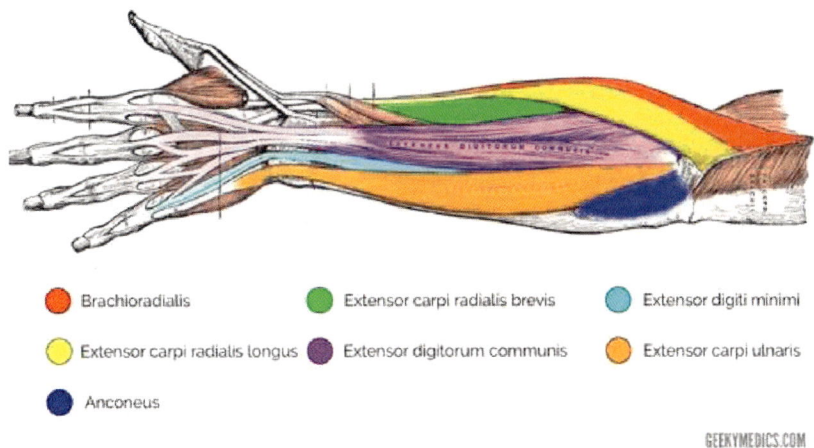

The superficial layer of the posterior compartment contains seven muscles that have a common origin of the supracondylar ridge and laterally epicondyle of the humerus (the common extensor tendon):

- Brachioradialis
- Extensor carpi radialis longus
- Extensor carpi radialis brevis
- Extensor digitorum
- Extensor digiti minimi
- Extensor carpi ulnaris

https://geekymedics.com/muscles-of-the-posterior-forearm

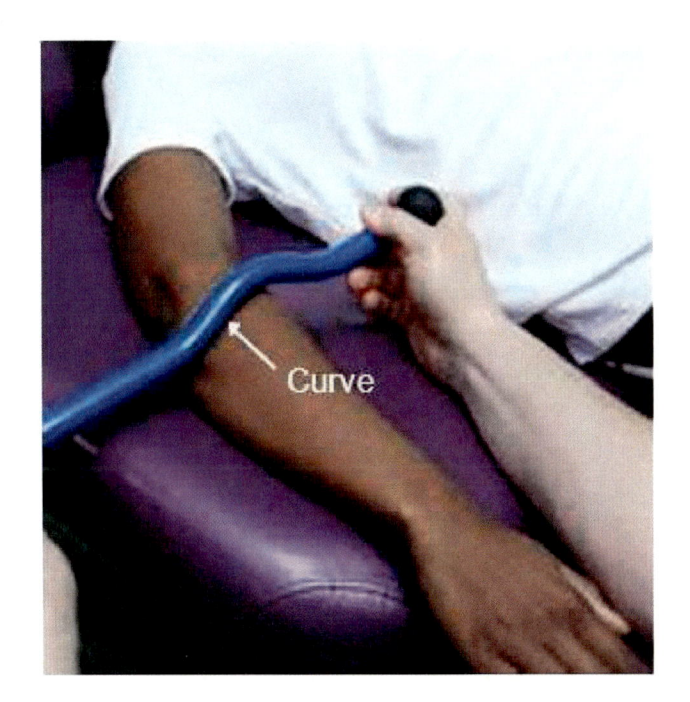

LUBRICATION: None

TPRT:

Curve

Anterior Forearm – Curve

TECHNIQUE MOTION:

Place TPRT on posterior forearm and engage the tissues with the Curve. <u>Do not slide</u> the TPRT. Move the tissue in a small circle or up and down.

TPRT™ MODULE 4 – CLIENT THERAPY

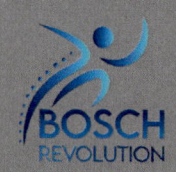

EDUCATION:

Biceps Brachii - Brachialis

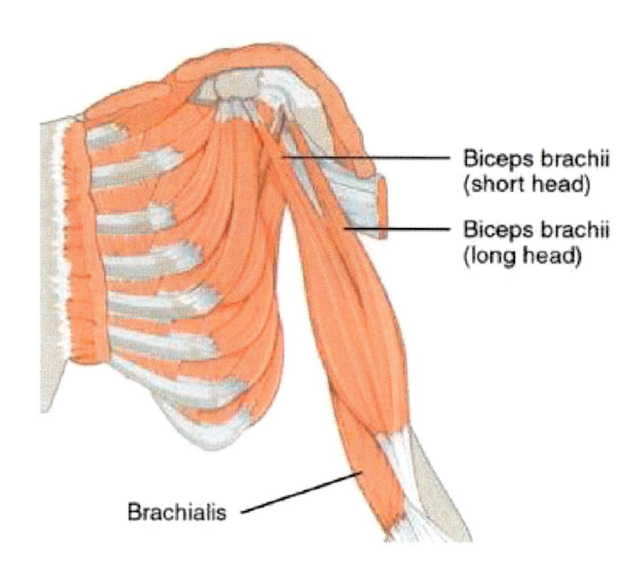

https://upload.wikimedia.org/wikipedia/commons/3/36/1120_Muscles_that_Move_the_Forearm_Humerus_Flex_Sin.png

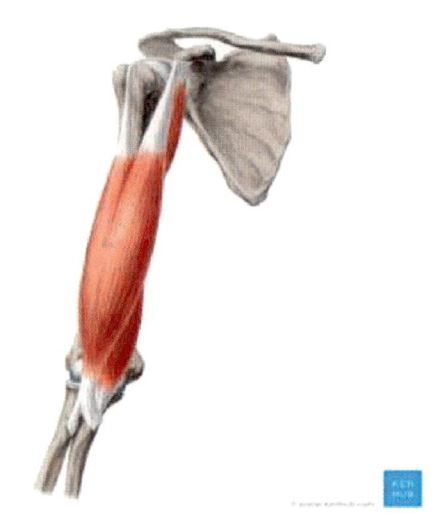

https://www.kenhub.com/thumbor/b0BpruXM7o46A10JLNgrvjPr26s=/fit-in/800x1600/filters:watermark(/images/logo_url.png,-10,-10,0):background_color(FFFFFF):format(jpeg)/images/library/14494/518_biceps_brachii_coracobrachialis_brachialis_muscles_anterior_view_YK_copy.png

ARM RELEASE (SIDE LYING AND PRONE) - FLAT EDGE
BICEPS BRACII, BRACHIORADIALIS, AND BRACHIALIS

LUBRICATION: None

TPRT:
Flat Edge

TECHNIQUE MOTION:

Flat Edge: Use the flat edge to engage the tissues of the Anterior Biceps and pivot or move in a circular motion. Apply pressure on the exhale.

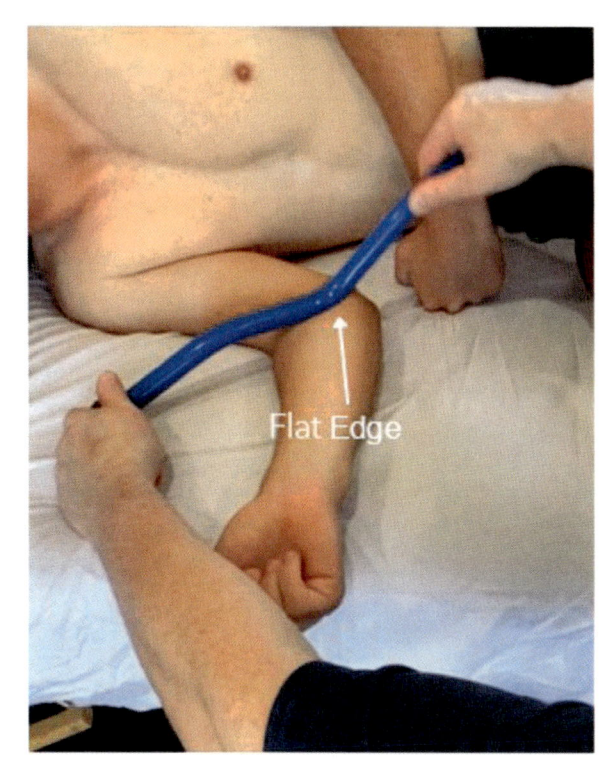

Arm Release – Edge

Slope: Use the Slope to engage the Posterior Biceps Bracii, Brachioradialis and Brachialis. Pivot the Slope or move it in a circular direction.

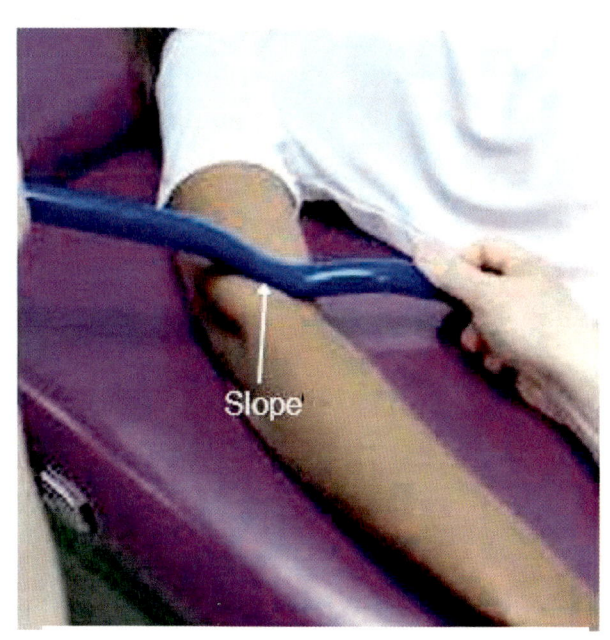

Arm Release - Slope

ARM RELEASE: MIDDLE BICEPS BRACHII - CURVE AND SLOPE

LUBRICATION: Oil or Lotion

TPRT:
Curve and Slope

TECHNIQUE MOTION:

Curve: Begin just above the proximal elbow and slide the Curve up and down. Have the client breathe in for 3 seconds and slowly exhale. Slide the TPRT up the arm.

Slope: Use the Curve to engage the Biceps Bracii, Brachioradialis, and Brachialis. Pivot the Curve or move it in a circular direction.

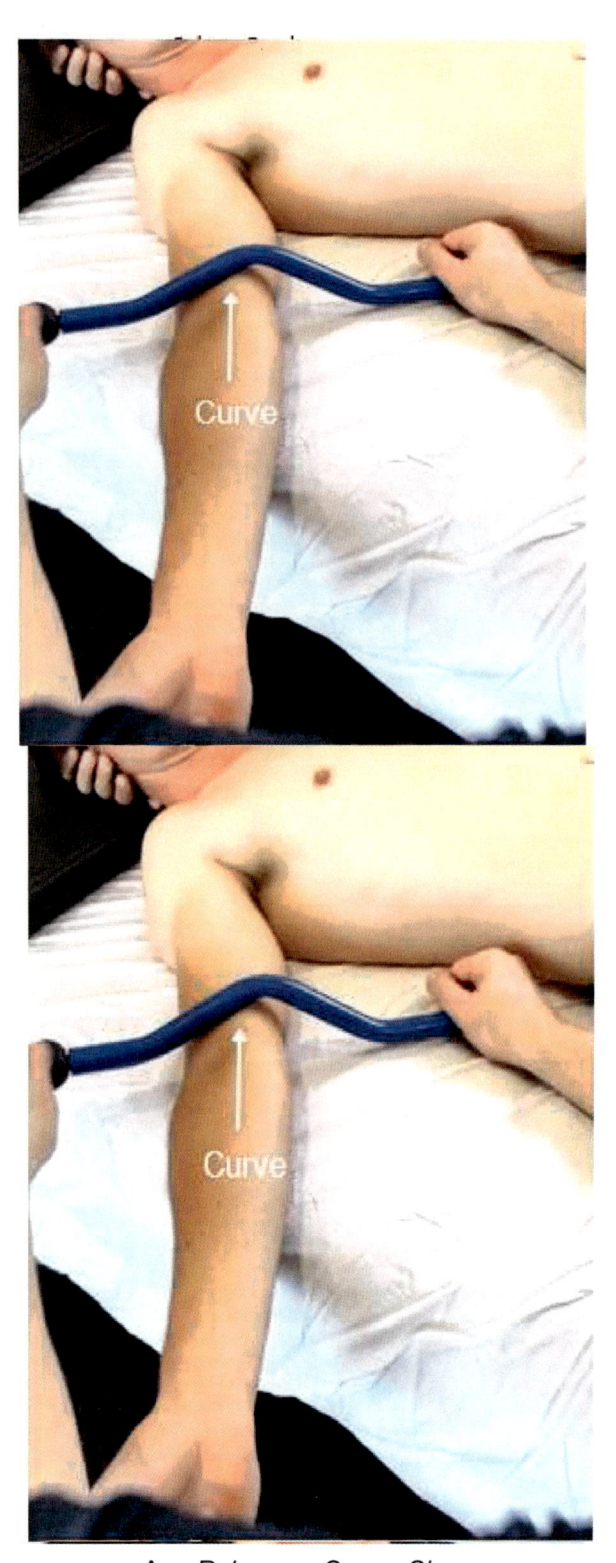

Arm Release – Curve, Slope

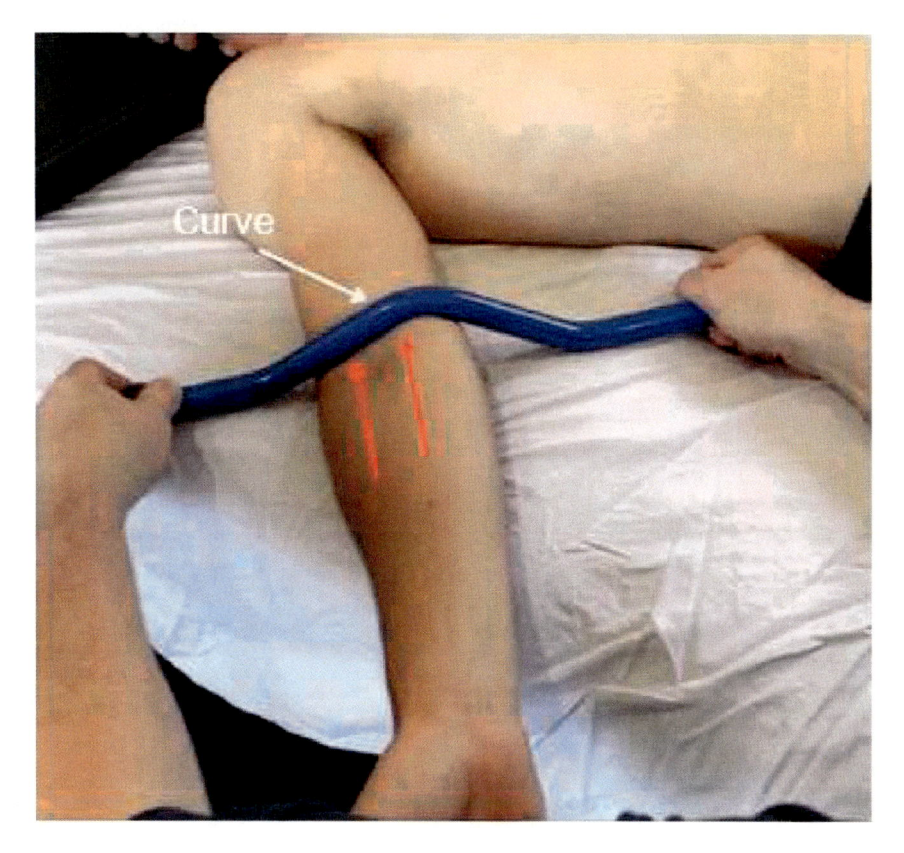

DISTAL BICEPS RELEASE - CURVE

Distal Biceps Release – Curve

LUBRICATION:
Oil or Lotion to anterior biceps

TPRT:
Curve

TECHNIQUE MOTION:
Curve: Use the Curve to lightly engage the tissue of the anterior biceps. Engage the muscle and move back and forth, from side to side and up and down. Apply pressure on the exhale.

Do this for 15 to 30 seconds.

TPRT MODULE 4 – CLIENT THERAPY

EDUCATION:

POSTERIOR ROTATOR CUFF & TRICEPS

1. Supraspinatus
2. Posterior Deltoid
3. Infraspinatus
4. Teres Minor
5. Teres Major
6. Triceps
7. Latissimus Dorsi

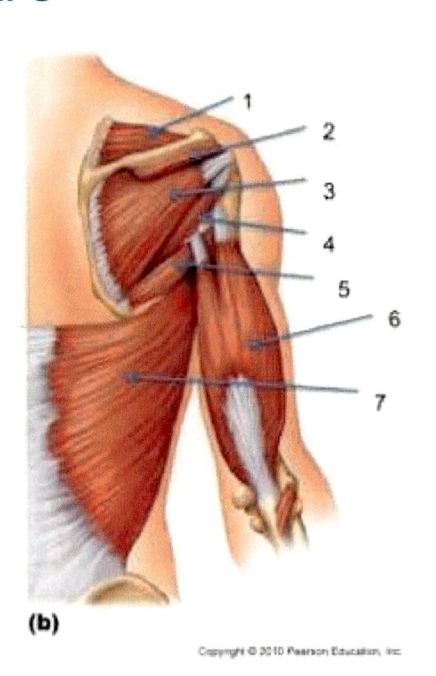

Triceps Brachii Trigger Points

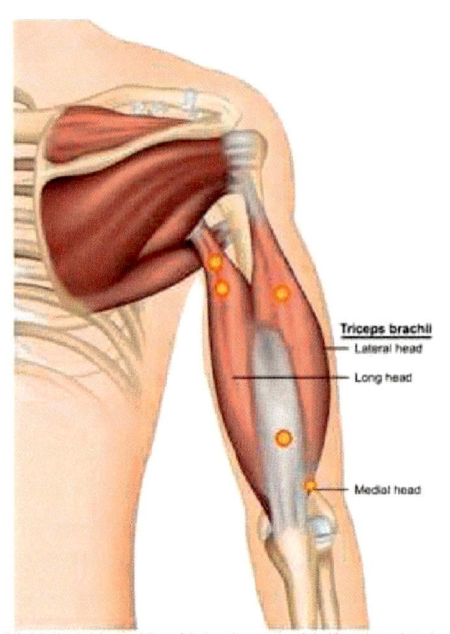

The triceps brachii is a three headed muscle which connects the shoulder blade (scapula) and the upper arm (humerus) to the lower arm (ulna). The muscle is found in the back of the upper arm.

https://thewellnessdigest.com/wp-content/uploads/2013/03/triceps-brachii-trp.jpg

TRICEPS AND SERRATUS ANTERIOR RELEASE – CURVE & SMALL KNOB

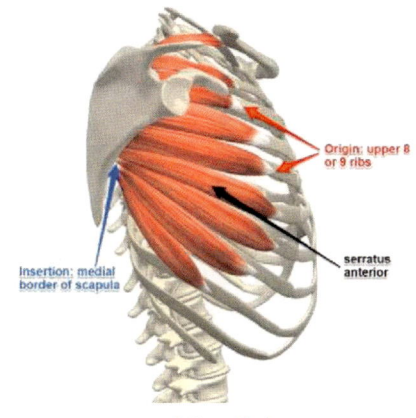

https://cdn-aolkg.nitrocdn.com/JEsNUzsMoDdLghSXkopLhNFWnBniacqf/assets/images/optimized/rev-4af294e/wp-content/uploads/2020/08/serratus-anterior-muscle.jpg

LUBRICATION: Oil or Lotion to triceps

TPRT:
Curve

TECHNIQUE MOTION:
<u>Slide</u> the Curve up and down the triceps muscle.

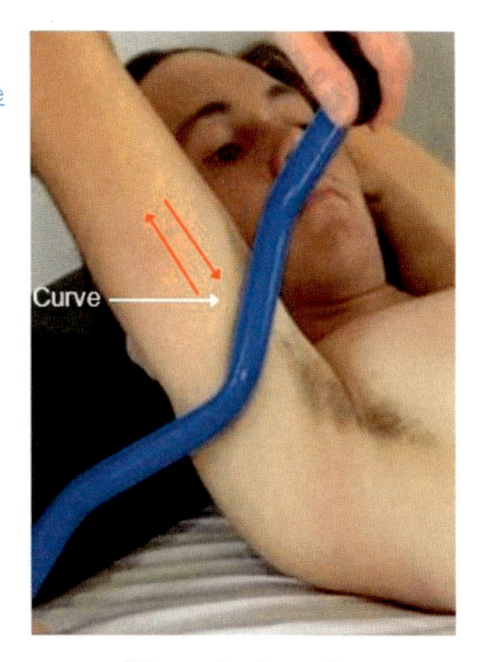

Triceps Supine – Curve

SERRATUS ANTERIOR RELEASE (SUPINE)

LUBRICATION: None

TPRT:
Small Knob

TECHNIQUE MOTION:
Place the knob on the Serratus Anterior and <u>rock back and forth</u> gently.

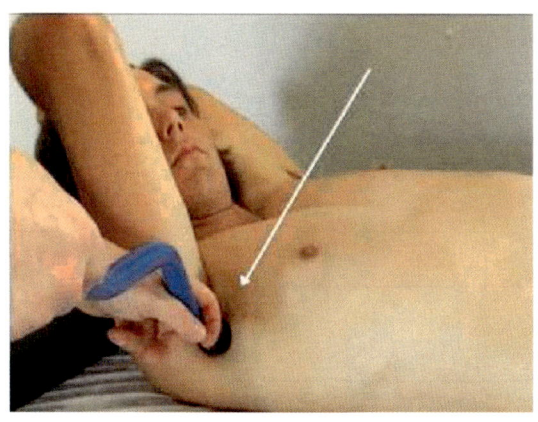

Serratus Anterior Release Supine – Small Knob

TRICEPS RELEASE (PRONE) - CURVE

Triceps Brachii Long Head & Lateral Head, Triceps Brachii Tendon

LUBRICATION: Oil or Lotion

TPRT:

Curve

TECHNIQUE MOTION:

Place Curve and the V of TPRT on the triceps just above the elbow.

Slide up the arm.

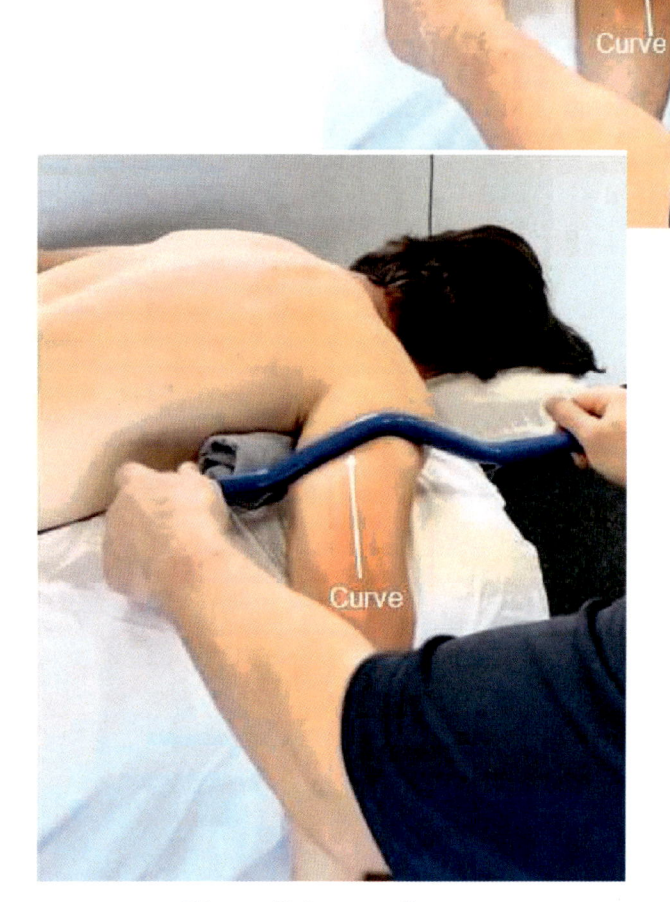

Triceps Release – Curve

SHOULDER RELEASE (PRONE) - CURVE

Release Infraspinatus Muscle

LUBRICATION: Oil or Lotion

TPRT:

Small Knob

TECHNIQUE MOTION:

Have the client breathe in as they exhale to a five-count, and you will apply pressure to release the posterior shoulder.

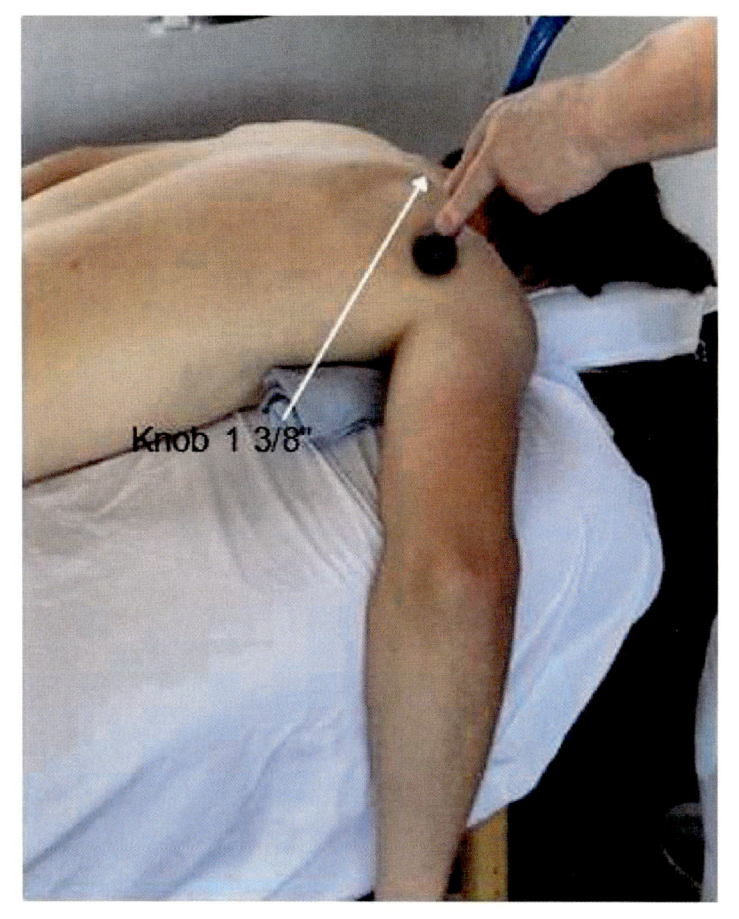

Shoulder Release – Curve

TPRT™ MODULE 5 – CLIENT THERAPY

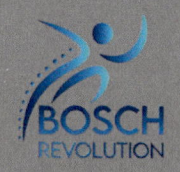

FOOT RELEASE PART 1 - SMALL KNOB

LUBRICATION: None

TPRT:
Small Knob

TECHNIQUE MOTION:

Slide the Knob up and down.

Move the Knob in a <u>circular direction</u>.

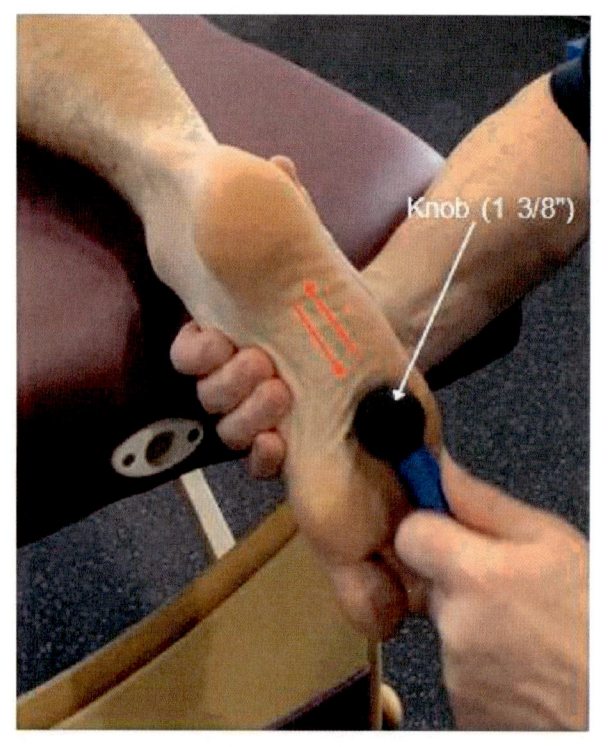

Foot Release – Small Knob

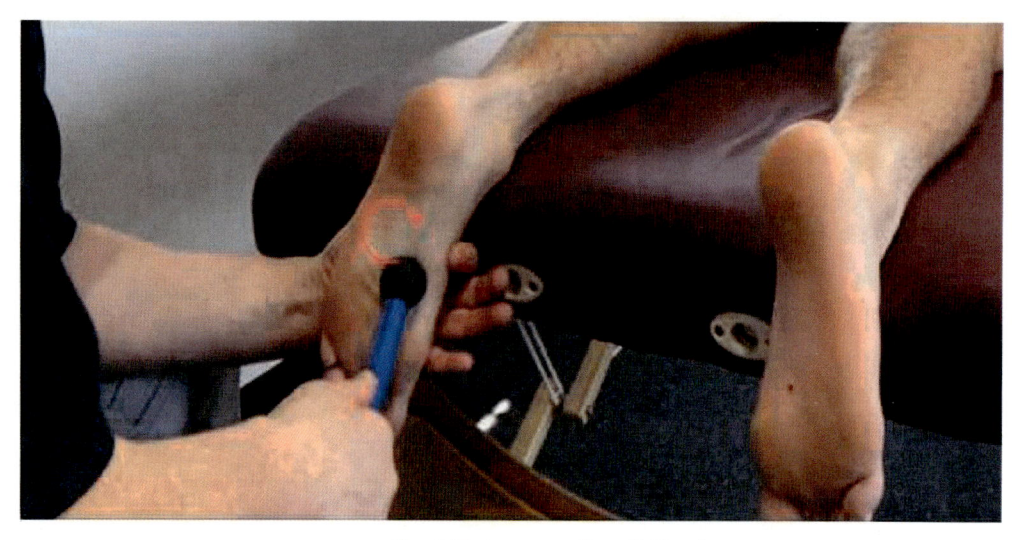

Foot Release – Small Knob

TPRT MODULE 5 – CLIENT THERAPY

FOOT RELEASE PART 2 - SMALL KNOB

LUBRICATION: With or without Oil or Lotion

TPRT:

Small Knob

TECHNIQUE MOTION:

Use the knob to release the bottom of the foot. Engage the muscles on the bottom of the foot and slowly pull down the foot. As you slide the knob between the metatarsal, be sure the pressure is okay with your client.

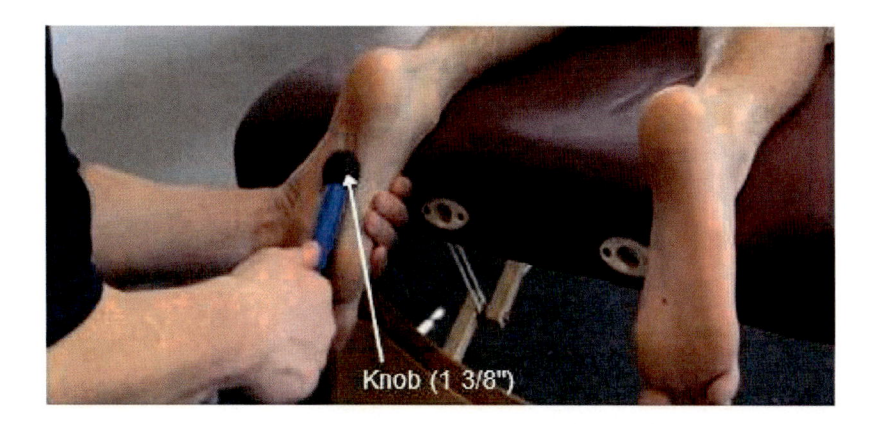

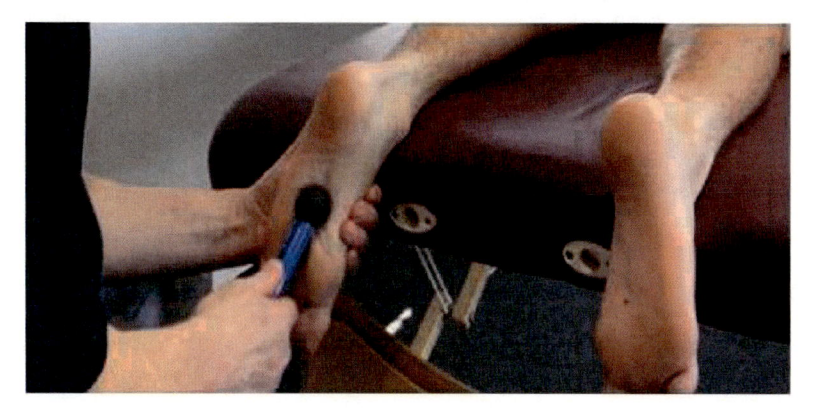

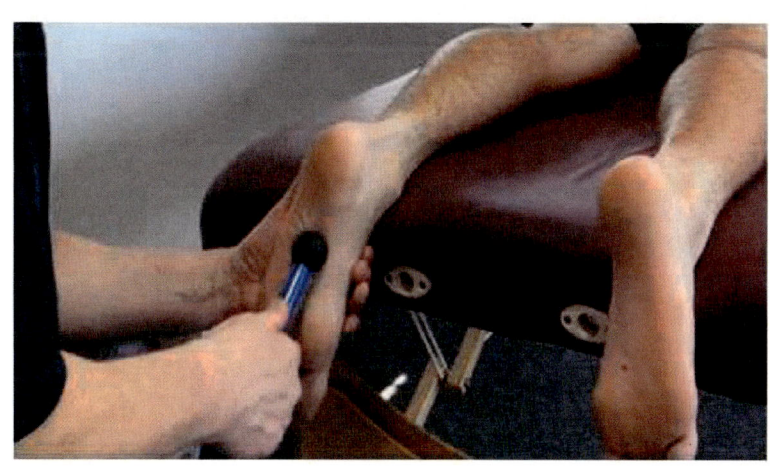

Knob (1 3/8")

Foot Release – Small Knob

59

TPRT MODULE 5 – CLIENT THERAPY

FOOT RELEASE PART 1 & 2 - SLOPE AND FLAT EDGE

PART 1

LUBRICATION: With or without a light amount of Oil or Lotion

TPRT:
Slope

TECHNIQUE MOTION:
Use the Slope to slide up and down the foot.

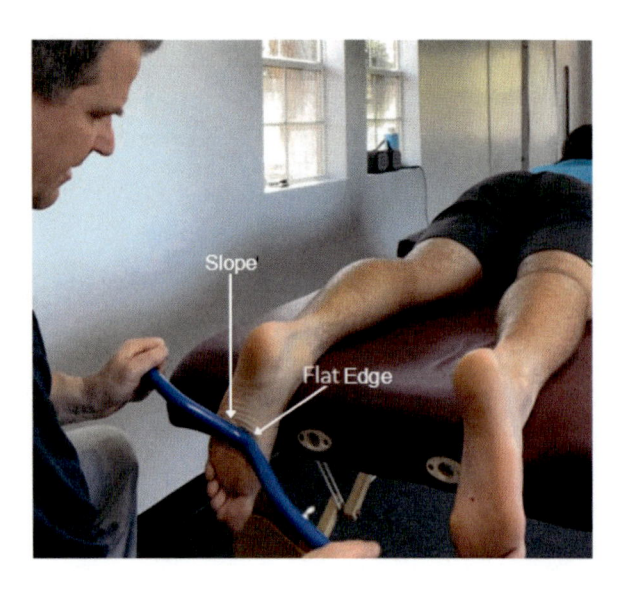

PART 2

TPRT:
Flat Edge

TECHNIQUE MOTION:
Place the Flat Edge on the heel. <u>Pivot back and forth</u>. Apply pressure on the exhale.

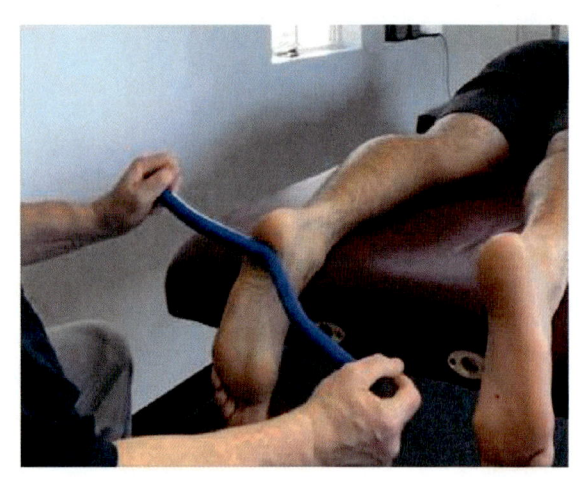

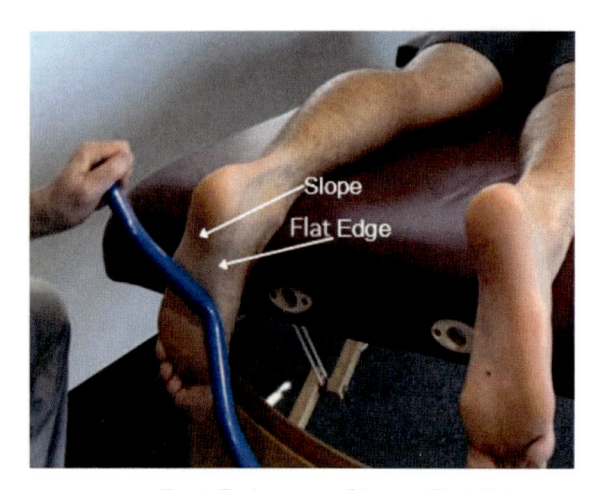

Foot Release – Slope, Flat Edge

TPRT MODULE 5 – CLIENT THERAPY

MEDIAL (INSIDE) CALF RELEASE - CURVE

LUBRICATION: Oil or Lotion

TPRT:

Curve

TECHNIQUE MOTION:

Spread the lotion with the TPRT. <u>Slide</u> it up the calf using the Curve.

Remember to stay off the shin bone when sliding up the calf.

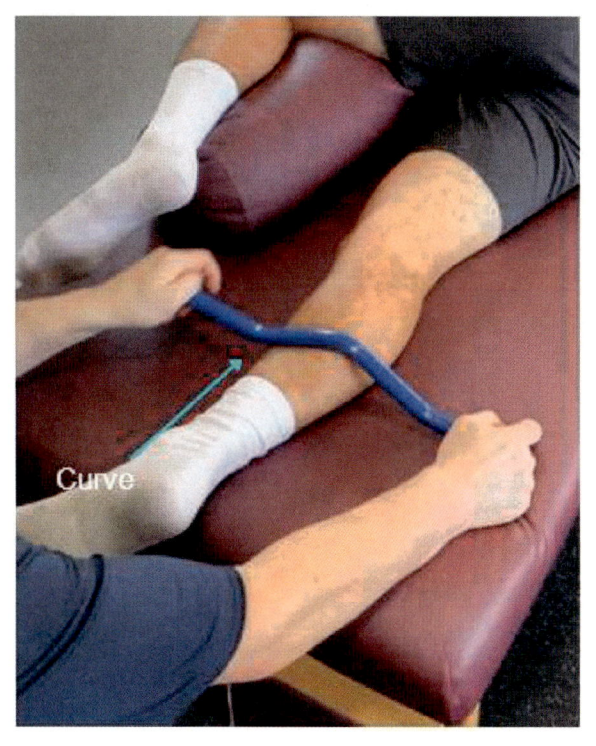

Inside Calf – Curve

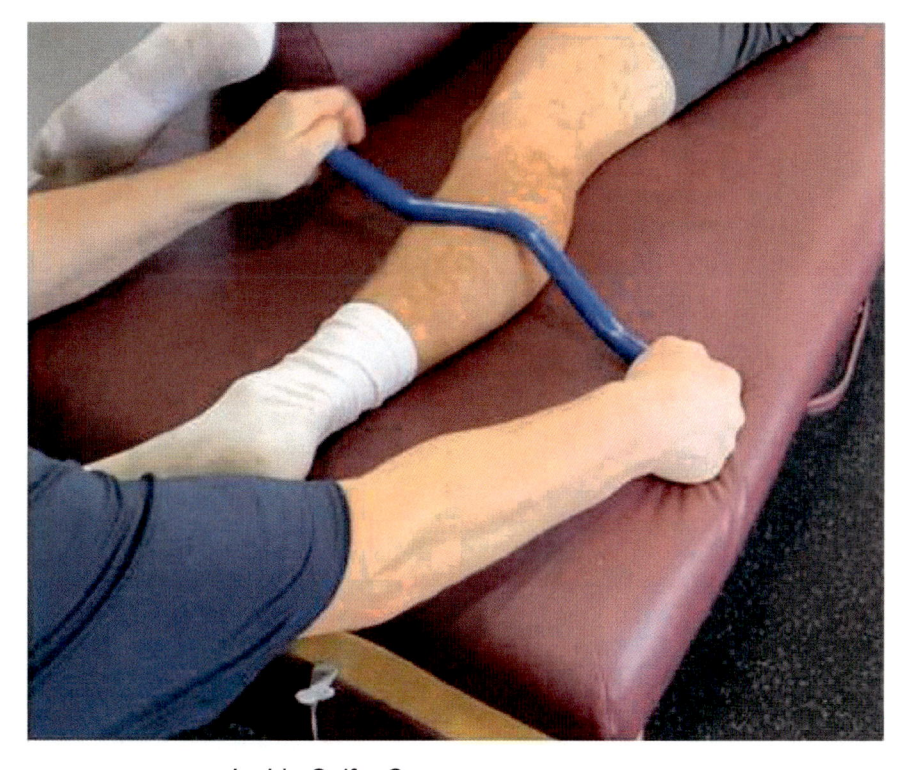

Inside Calf – Curve

61

TPRT MODULE 5 – CLIENT THERAPY

LATERAL (OUTSIDE) CALF RELEASE PART 1 - CURVE

LUBRICATION: Oil or Lotion

TPRT:
Curve

TECHNIQUE MOTION:

Use the Curve to slide down the outside of the calf.

Remember, do not put direct pressure on the tibia bone. Stay on the Tibialis Anterior muscle.

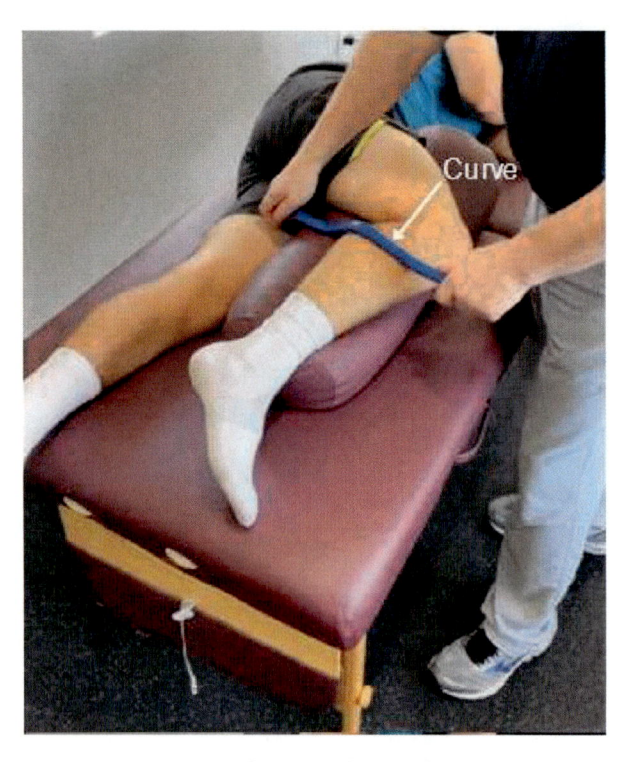

Outside Calf – Curve

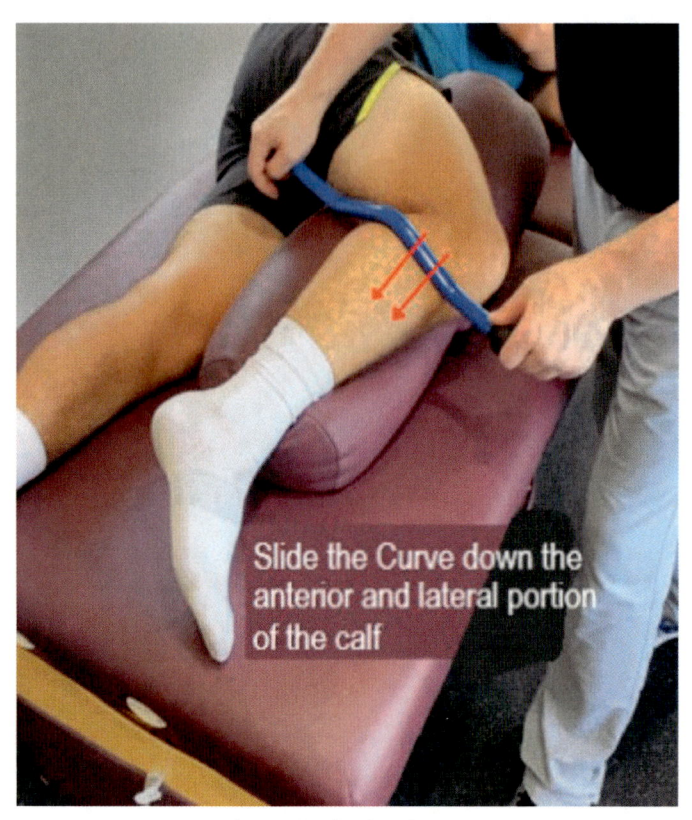

Outside Calf – Curve

LATERAL (OUTSIDE) CALF RELEASE PART 2 - CURVE

TIBIALIS ANTERIOR, EXTENSOR DIGITORUM LONGUS

LUBRICATION: Oil or Lotion

TPRT:
Curve

TECHNIQUE MOTION:
Slide the Curve down the lateral (outside) calf.

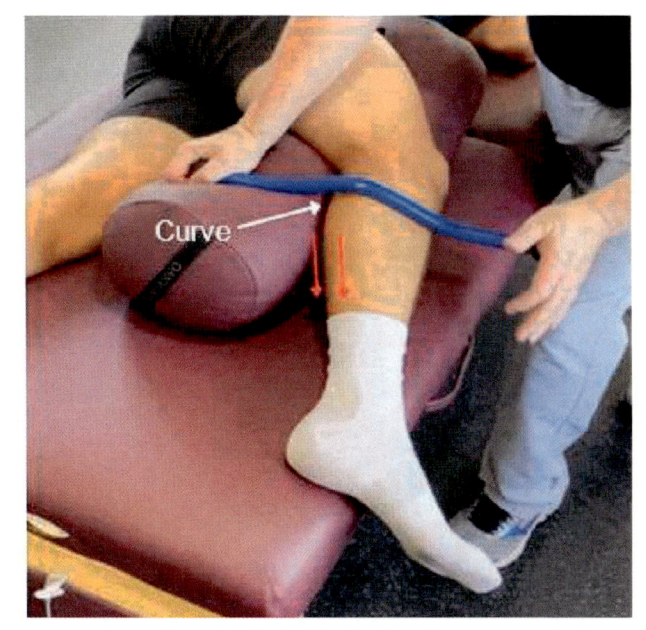

Lateral Outside Calf – Curve

Use Point 2 on the TPRT to release the Extensor Hallucis Longus.

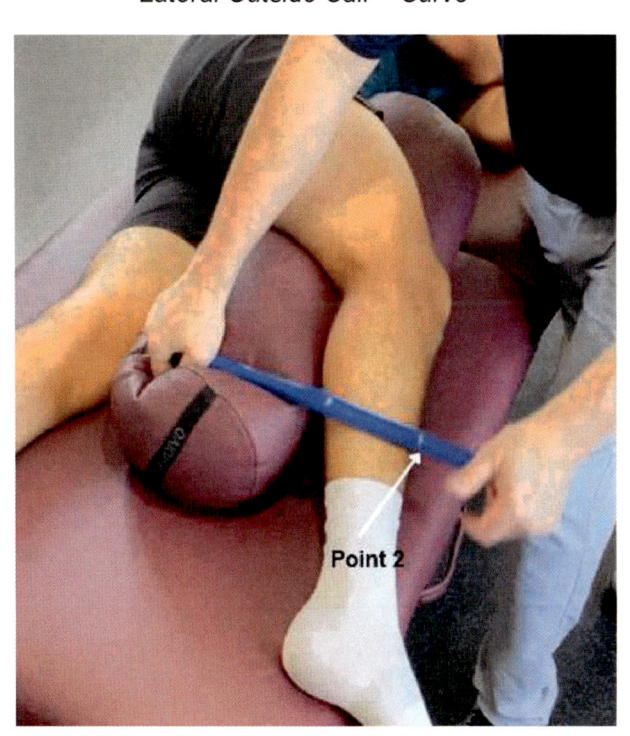

Lateral Outside Calf – Curve

CALF RELEASE: GASTROC (PRONE) – V & CURVES

CALF: ACHILLES, TENDON, AND LATERAL GASTROCNEMIUS

LUBRICATION: Oil or Lotion

TPRT:
V and Curves

TECHNIQUE MOTION:
Slide the V and the Curves up the outside of the calf.

Then, slide the TPRT over and use the Curve to release the outside part of the calf (Lateral Head of the Gastrocnemius).

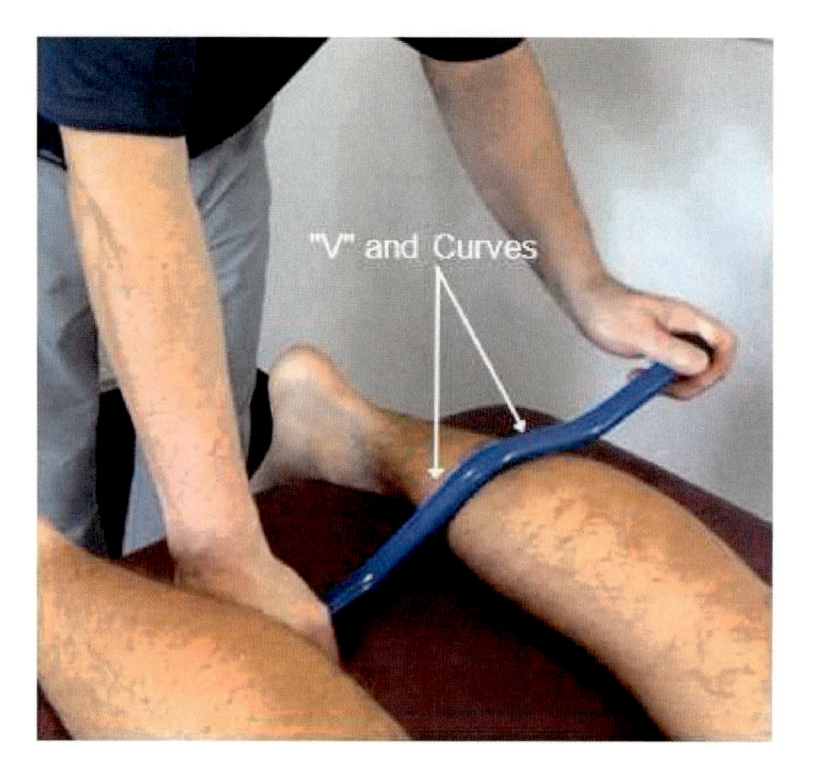

Calf Release – V, Curves

HOW TO RELEASE THE CALF (PRONE)

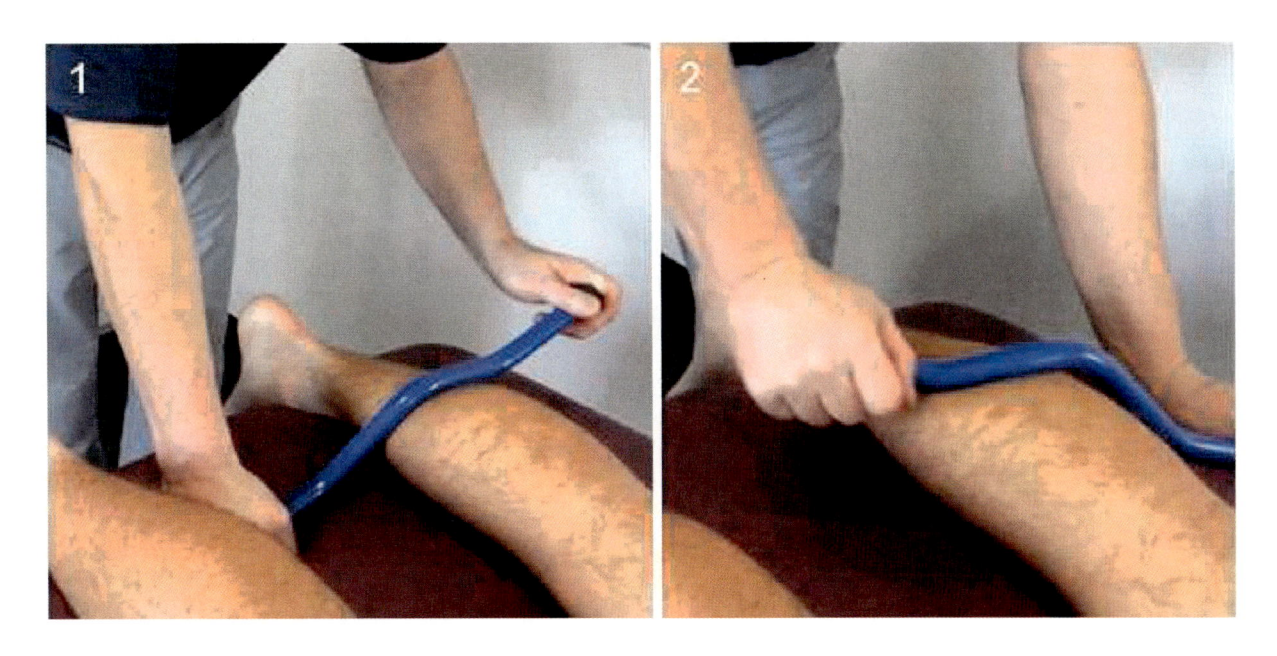

1. Use both Curves to slide up inner and outer calf.

2. Use the Curve to slide up the center of the calf.

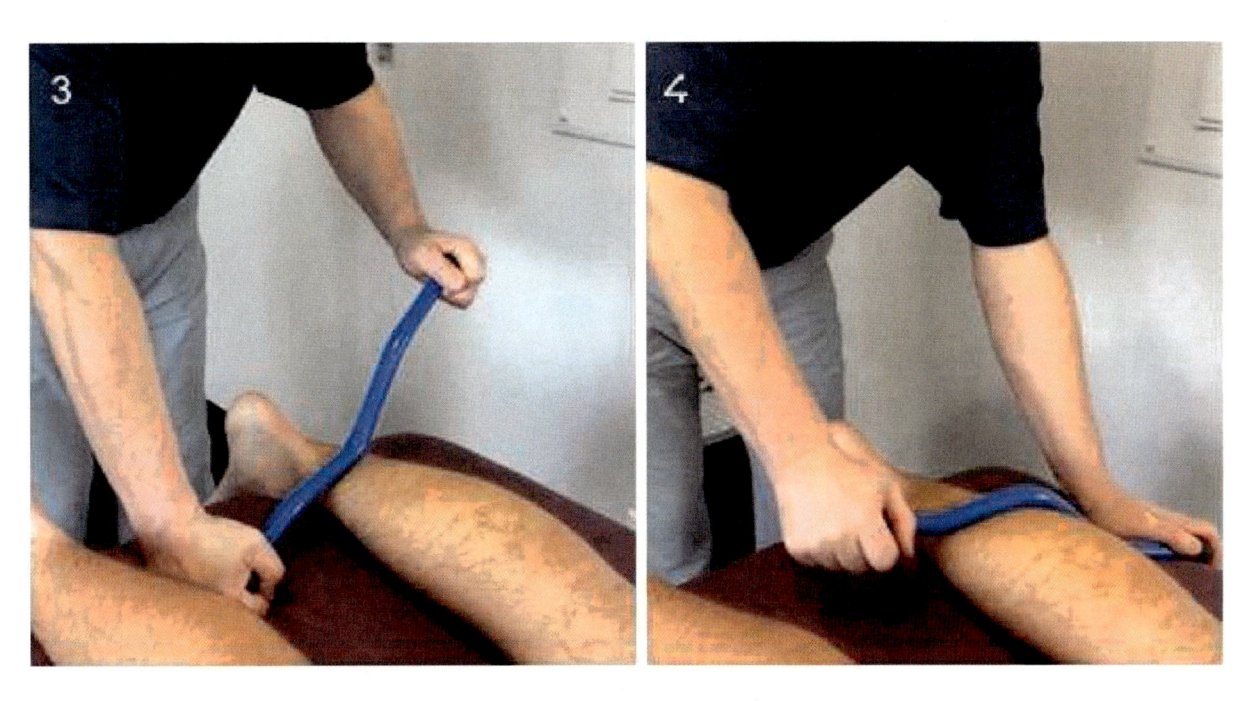

3. Use the Slope and Flat Edge to pin and pivot the TPRT over the lower portion of the calf

4. Use lotion and slide the Curve up the outside of the calf

TPRT™ MODULE 6 – CLIENT THERAPY

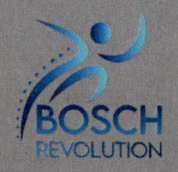

QUAD RELEASE - ABOVE KNEE (SEATED) – V & CURVES
RECTUS FEMORIS, VASTUS MEDIALIS, AND LATERALIS

LUBRICATION: Oil or Lotion

TPRT:
Slope, V, and Curves

TECHNIQUE MOTION:
Place the V just above (proximal) the knee.

Use the V and the 2 Slopes to slide the TPRT up the quad.

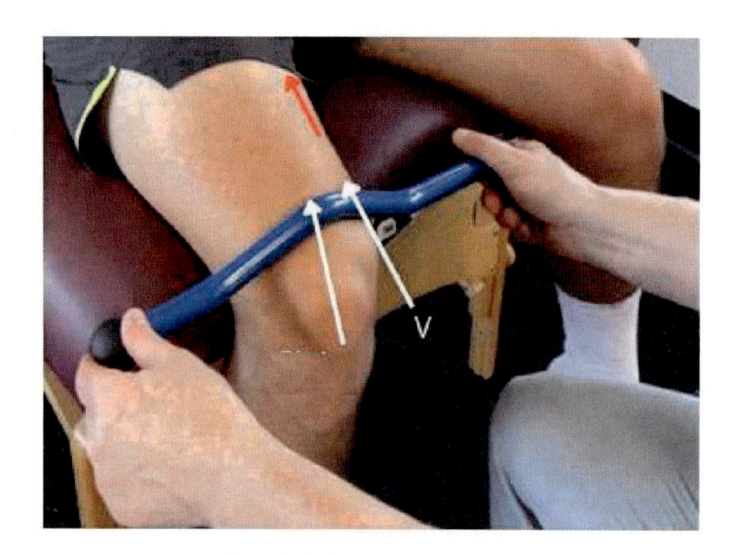

Quad Release – V

Slide the TPRT over to the side and use the Curve to slide up the quad.

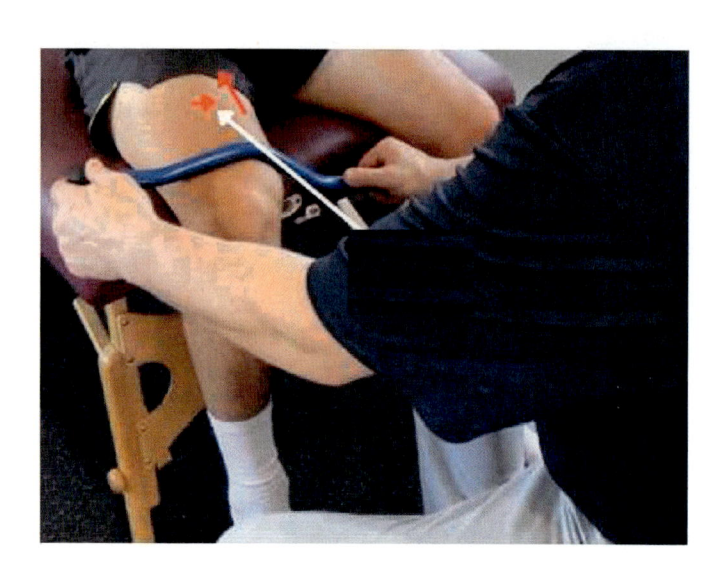

TPRT MODULE 6 – CLIENT THERAPY

IT BAND AND QUAD RELEASE (SEATED) – SLOPE, V & CURVES

IT BAND VASTUS LATERALIS WITH SLOPE

LUBRICATION: Oil or Lotion

TPRT:

Slope, V, and Curves

TECHNIQUE MOTION:

<u>Slide</u> up the IT Band with the Slope.

Use the V and the 2 Slopes to slide the TPRT up the quad.

Lower the outside hand to add more pressure to the IT Band. When you do this, you are using the Flat Edge portion of the tool.

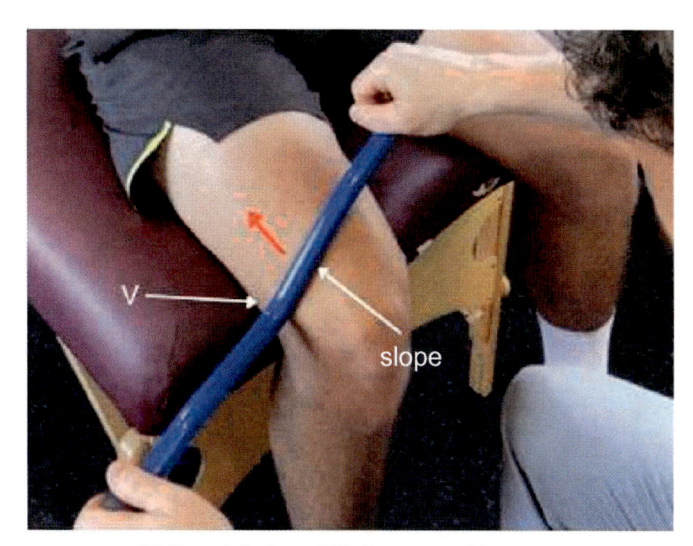

IT Band & Quad Release – Slope

VASTUS LATERALIS, RECTUS FEMORIS

TECHNIQUE MOTION:

<u>Slide</u> up the quad muscle using the Curve.

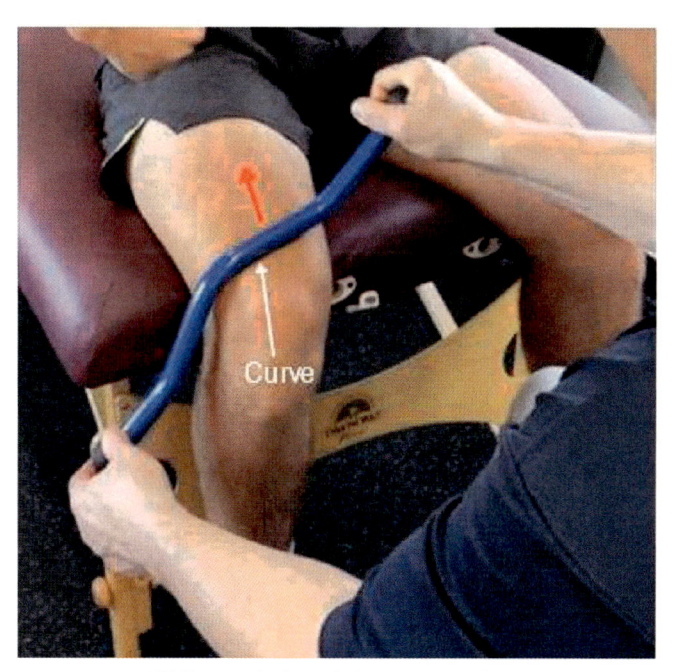

IT Band & Quad Release – Curves

67

TPRT MODULE 6 – CLIENT THERAPY

PATELLA RELEASE (SEATED)

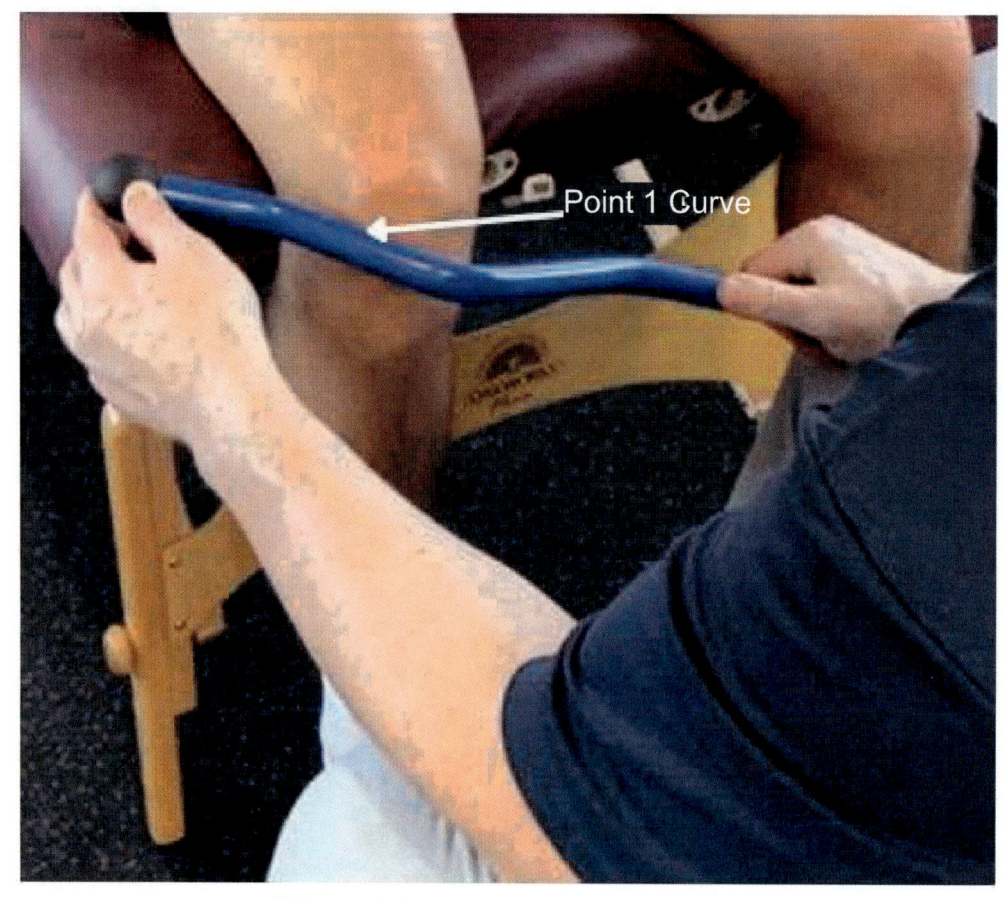

IT Band & Quad Release – Curve & Point 1

LUBRICATION: With or without Oil

TPRT:

Curve and Point 1

TECHNIQUE MOTION:

Use the Curve to work around the knee.

Remember to go lightly around the knee.
To learn how it feels, begin by practicing on your own knee.

IT BAND RELEASE (SIDE LYING) PART 1 – CURVE

LUBRICATION: Oil or Lotion

TPRT:

Curve

TECHNIQUE MOTION:

Place the Curves just above the knee. Use the Curves to <u>slide</u> the TPRT up the IT Band and lateral Quad.

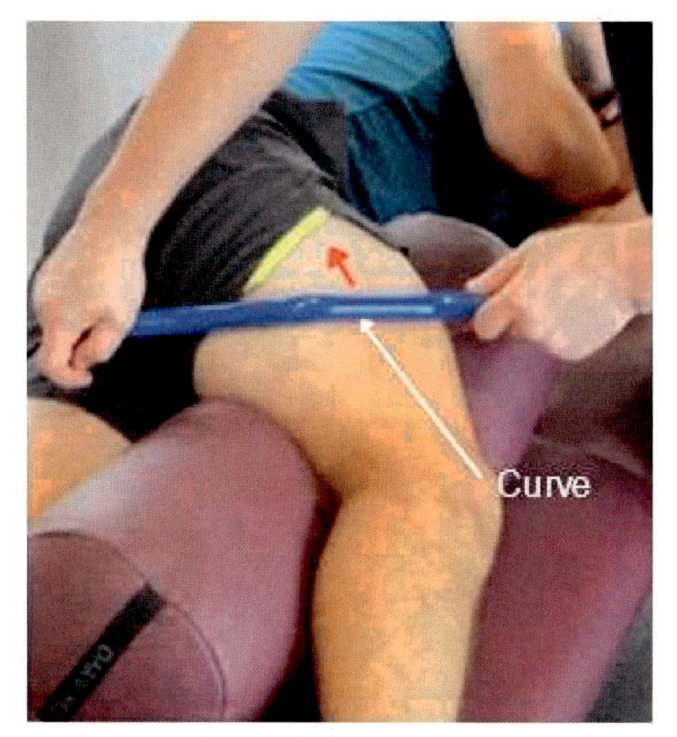

IT Band Release – Curves

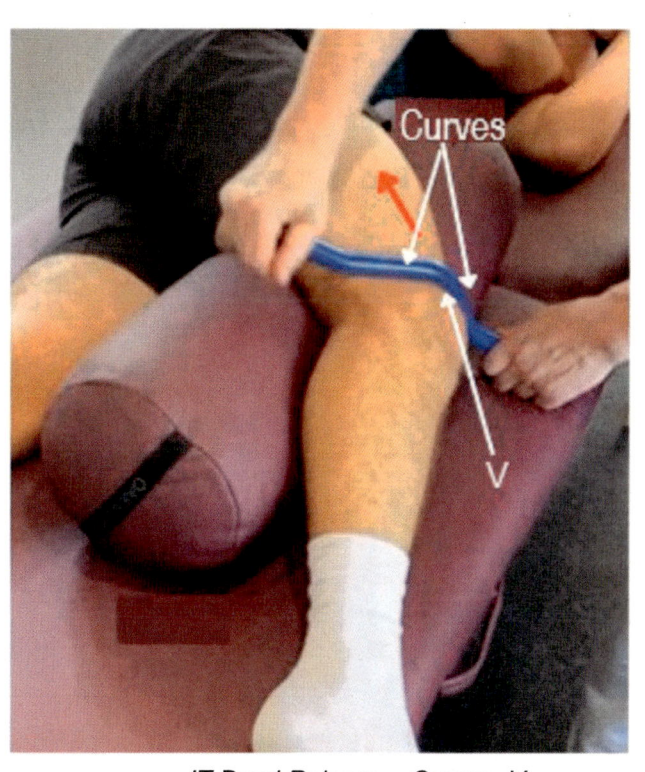

IT Band Release – Curves, V

TPRT MODULE 6 – CLIENT THERAPY

IT BAND RELEASE (SIDE LYING) PART 2 – CURVES

LUBRICATION: Oil or Lotion

TPRT:

Curves

TECHNIQUE MOTION:

Place the Curves on the IT Band just above the knee. <u>Slide</u> up the leg (IT Band).

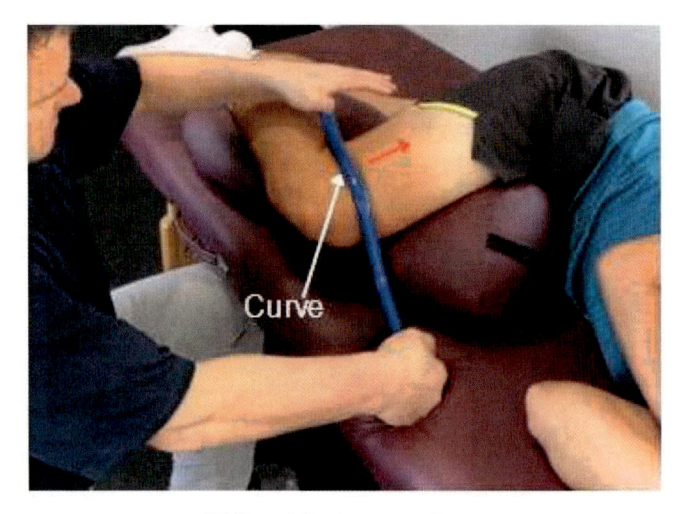

IT Band Release – Curves

Move the TPRT to the side (medial) and use the Curves to release the IT Band and Vastus Lateralis.

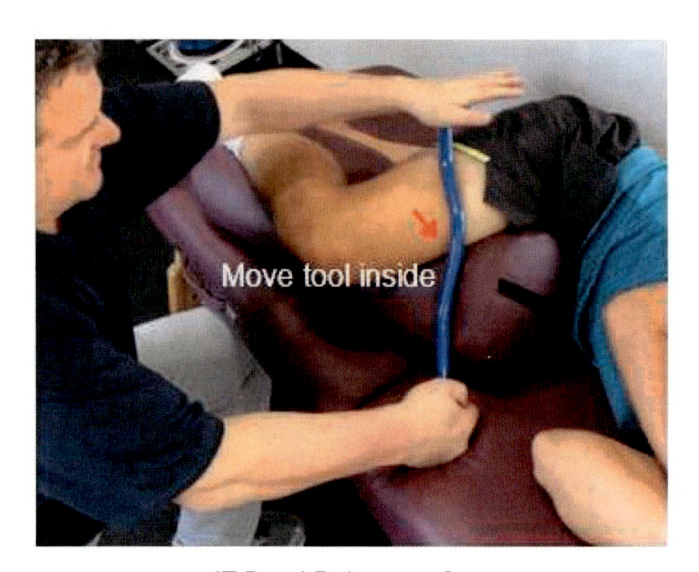

IT Band Release – Curves

ADDUCTOR RELEASE (INNER THIGH) – SLOPE & CURVE

LUBRICATION: Oil or Lotion

TPRT:

Curve and Slope

TECHNIQUE MOTION:

Beginning at the medial knee, use the Slope on the TPRT to slide up the leg. When you release the adductors, it is important to slide up the leg. This will have a cleansing effect on the body as you increase the venous return.

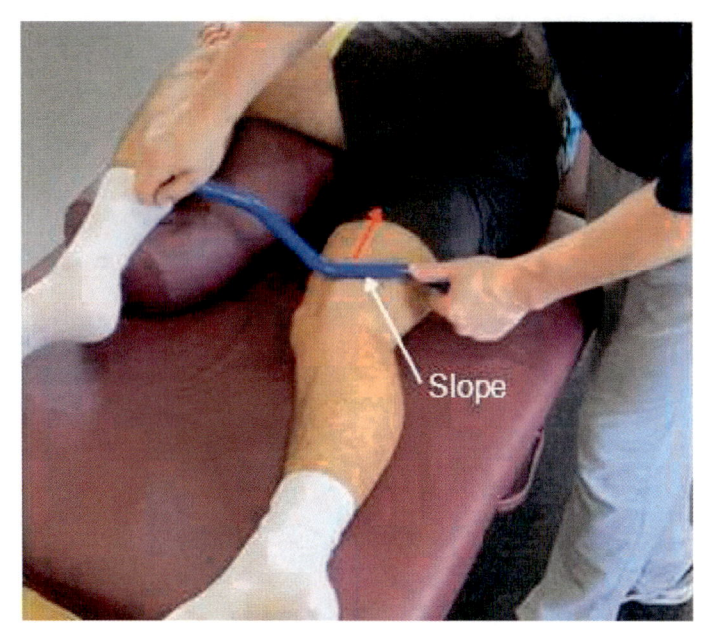

Adductor Release – Slope

Use the Curve to slide up (proximal) the leg from mid-thigh towards the ischial tuberosity.

Use the Curve to rock back and forth.

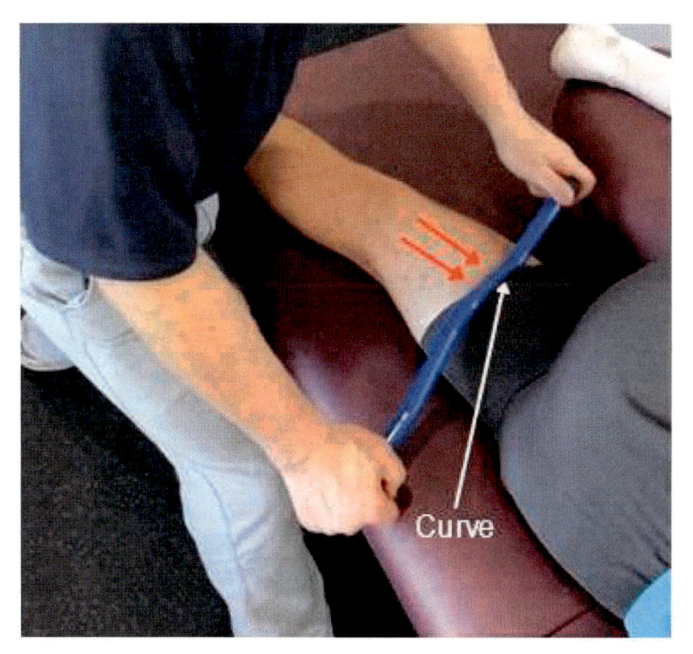

Adductor Release – Curve

PSOAS RELEASE

LUBRICATION:
None

TPRT:
Small Knob

TECHNIQUE MOTION:

Place the knob attachment on the inside (medial) of the inner thigh where the Psoas attaches to the Trochanter. Use the knob to move up and down, or side to side.

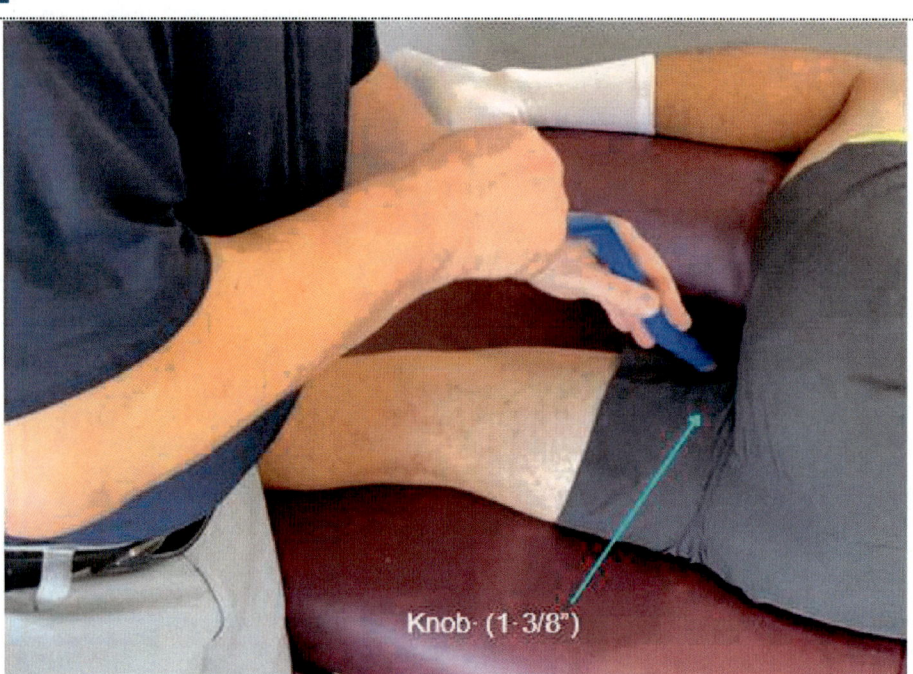

Knob- (1-3/8")

HAMSTRING RELEASE (PRONE) – SLOPE & FLAT EDGE

LUBRICATION: Oil or Lotion

TPRT:

Flat Edge and Slope

TECHNIQUE MOTION:

Place the Slope just above the proximal posterior knee and slide up the hamstring.

Move the TPRT to the side so the Flat Edge is in the middle of the hamstring.

Have the client breathe in. As they exhale, rock the tool back and forth to release the trigger points in the hamstrings.

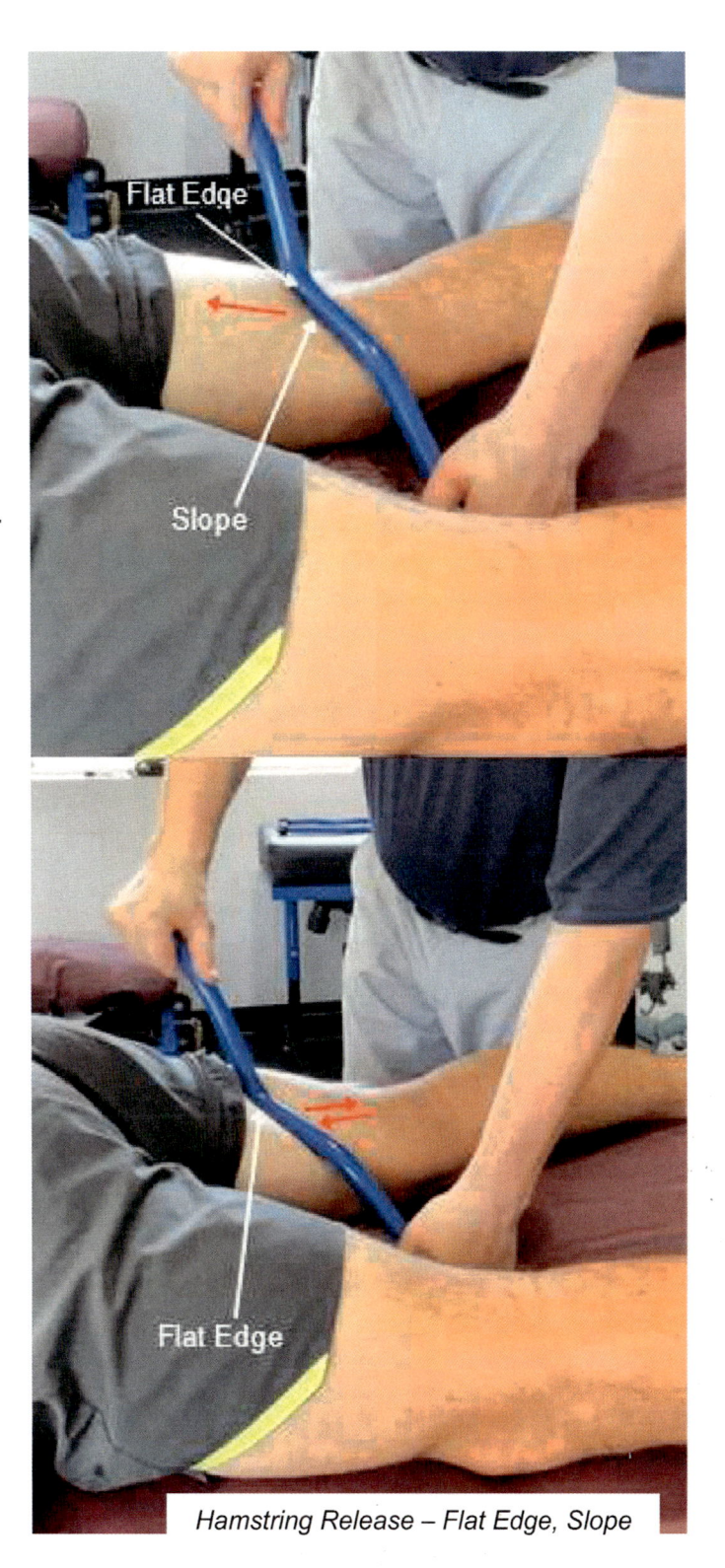

Hamstring Release – Flat Edge, Slope

HAMSTRING RELEASE (PRONE/SIDE-LYING) - SMALL KNOB

LUBRICATION: None

TPRT:

Small Knob

TECHNIQUE MOTION:

Place the knob just below the ischial tuberosity on the hamstring.

Have the client breathe in for 3 seconds, and as they exhale, apply pressure.

Ask the client how the pressure is and vary it to meet their satisfaction.

Work side to side or in a circular motion.

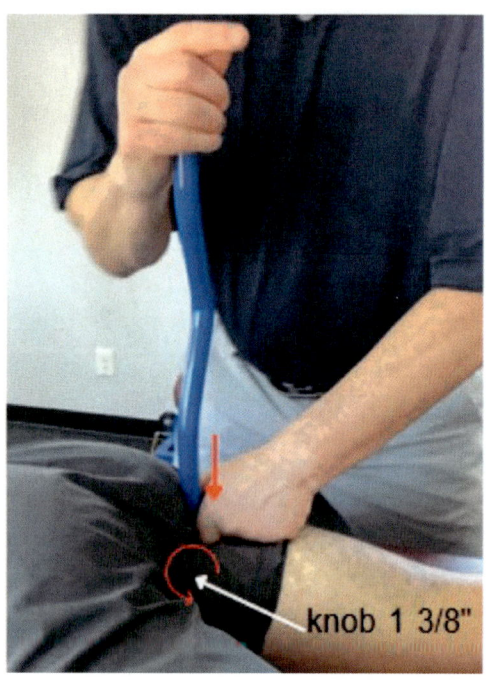

Hamstring Release – Small Knob

Hamstring Release – Small Knob

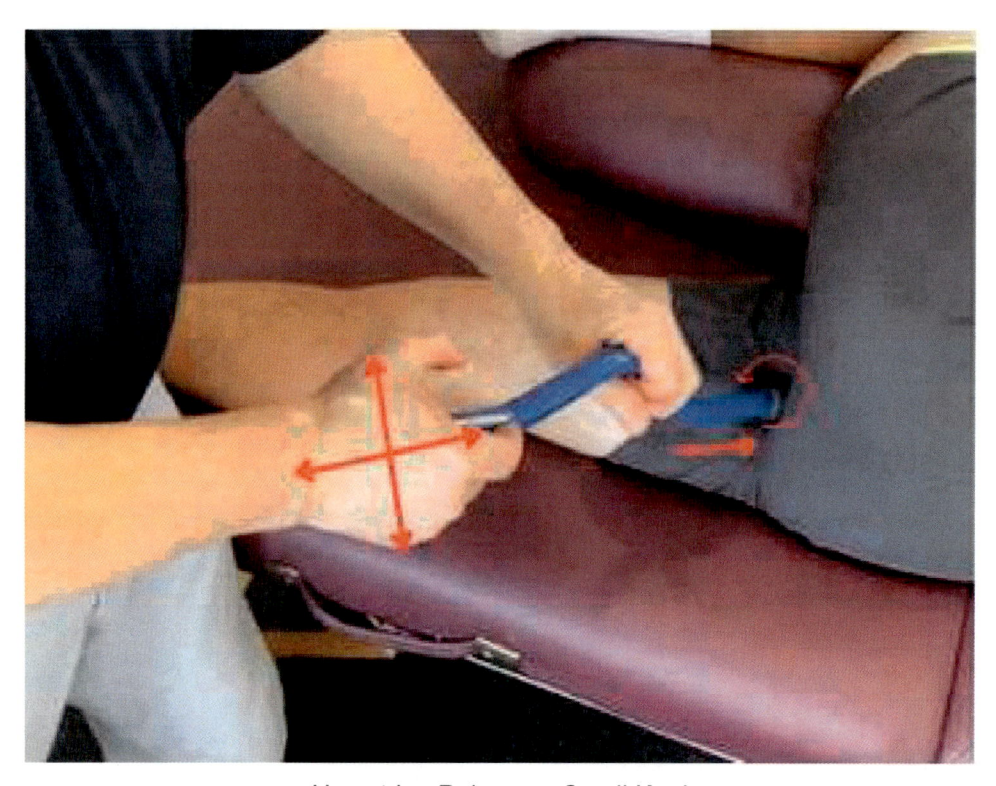

TPRT™ MODULE 7 – CLIENT THERAPY

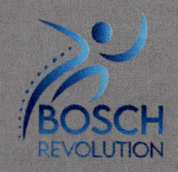

GLUTE MAX (PRONE) – CURVE

LUBRICATION: None

TPRT:
Curve

TECHNIQUE MOTION:
Use the Curve or slope to slide from the ilium down to the Trochanter.

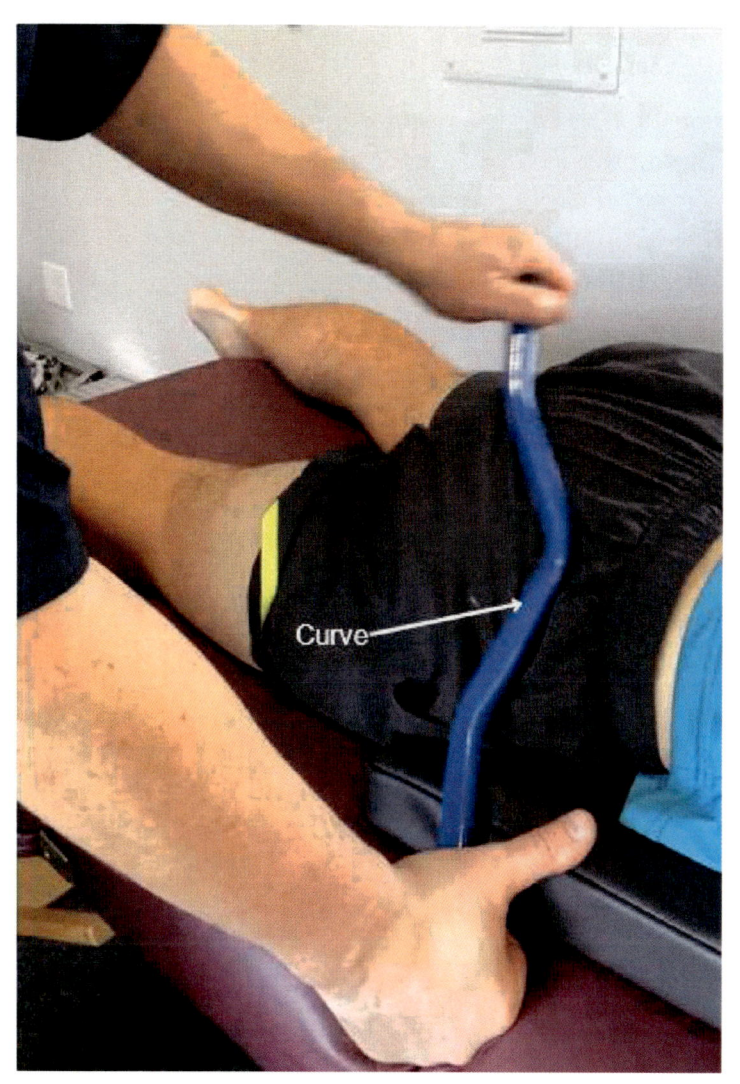

Glute Max Release – Curve

TPRT MODULE 7 – CLIENT THERAPY

GLUTE MEDIUS RELEASE - SMALL KNOB

LUBRICATION: None

TPRT:
Small Knob

TECHNIQUE MOTION:

Use your thumb to find the Greater Trochanter. Place the knob just above the (Superior Trochanter) work away from the Trochanter bone, down laterally into the fossa.

Place the top hand on the knob to move superior to inferior, and move away (superior or medially) from the bone.

Use your back hand to move laterally into the body. You can raise the back hand up and down to find different angles to work the TFL and glute medius muscles.

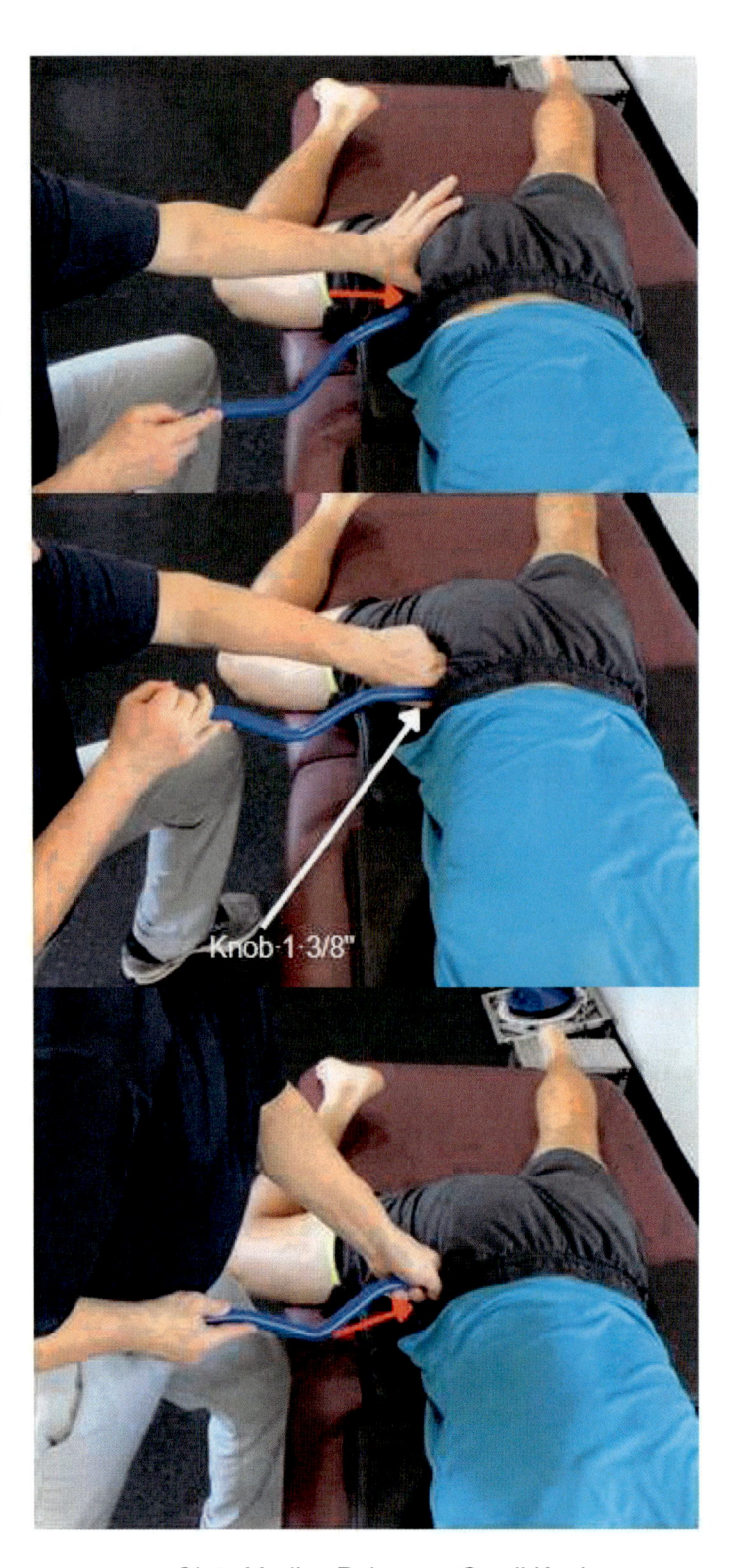

Glute Medius Release – Small Knob

GLUTE MEDIUS RELEASE (SIDE LYING) - SMALL KNOB & CURVE

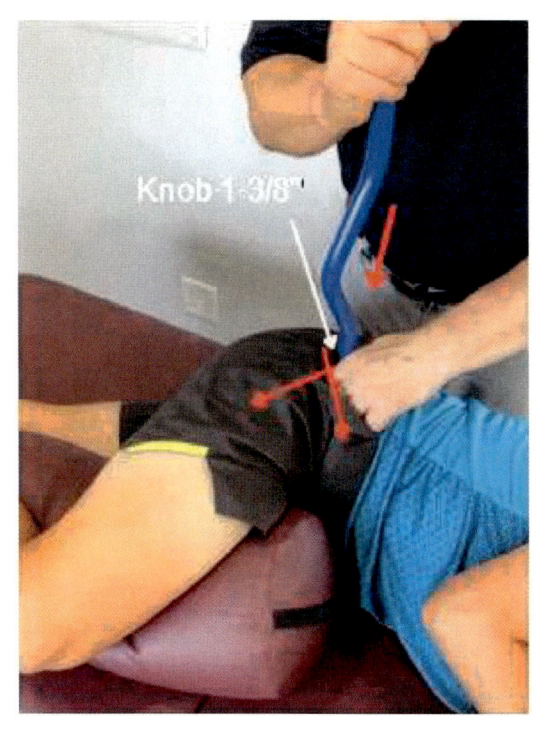

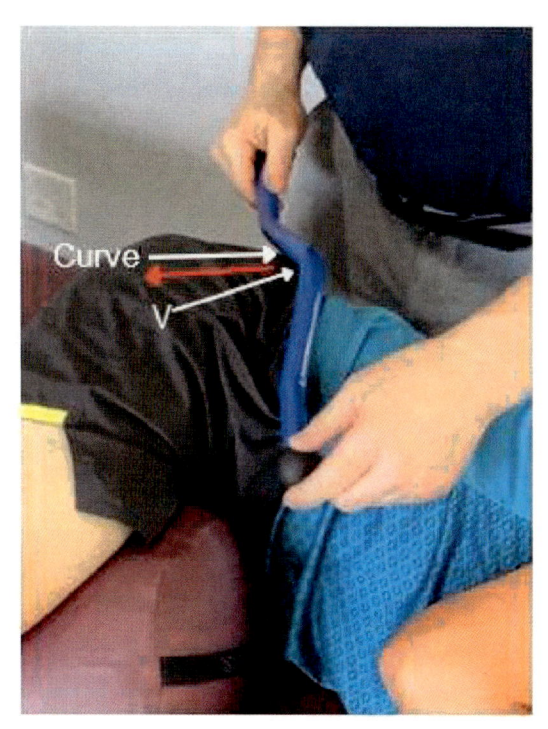

Glute Medius Release – Small Knob, Curve

LUBRICATION: None

TPRT:
Small Knob & Curve

TECHNIQUE MOTION:

Place the knob above the Trochanter. Stay off the bone and move medial to lateral and superior to inferior.

Place the Curves and the V just above the Trochanter. Engage and pin the gluteus medius and gluteus minimus muscles. Move from superior to inferior.

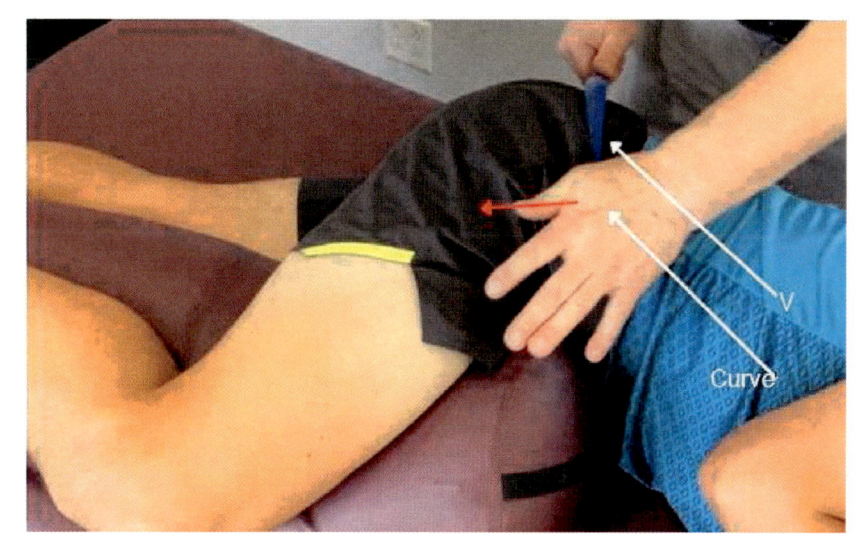

Glute Medius Release – Small Knob, Curve

Use your back hand to move laterally into the body. You can raise the back hand up and down to find different angles to work the TFL and glute medius muscles.

INTERNAL ROTATION ASSESSMENT - TFL RELEASE SMALL KNOB

Test Internal Hip Rotation 40°.

LUBRICATION: None

TPRT:

Small Knob

TECHNIQUE MOTION:

Place the knob distal to the Trochanter on the Tensor Fasciae latae. Move the knob up and down and side to side.

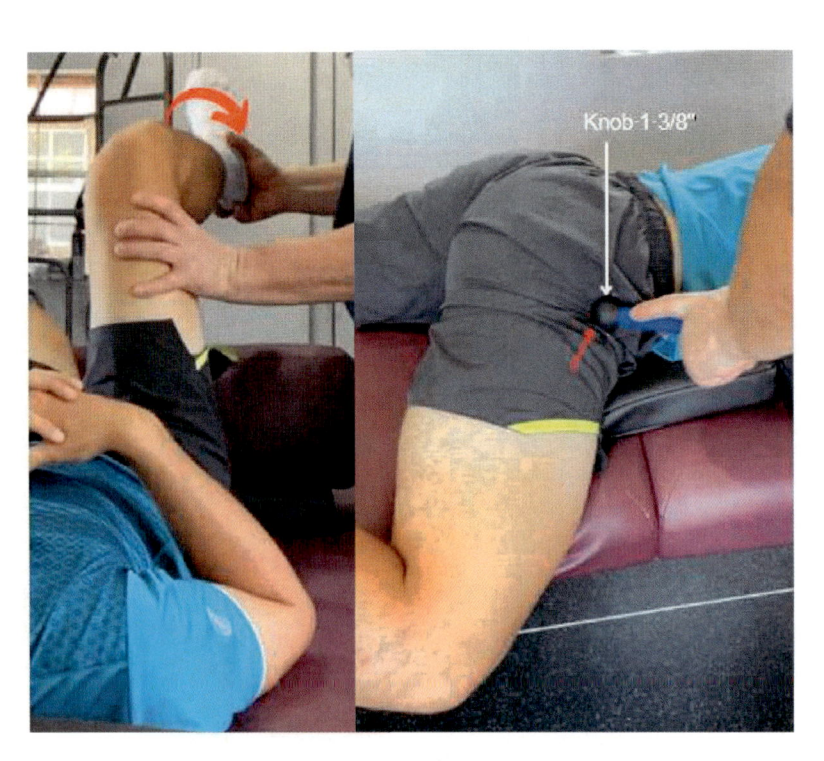

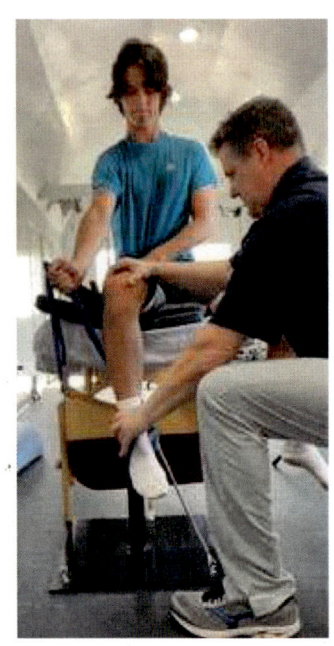

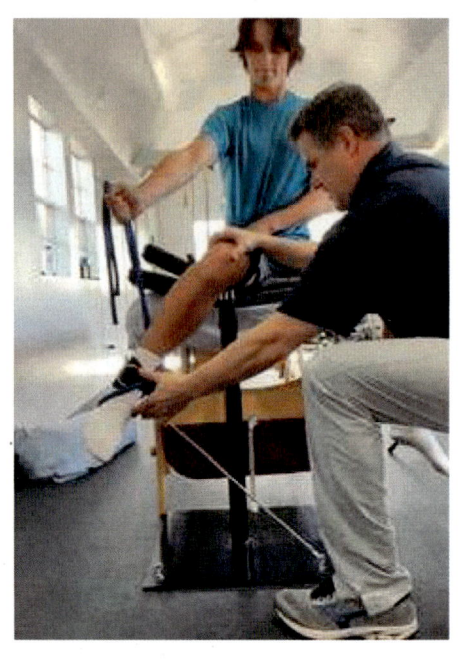

In the top left photo, this tennis player has no internal hip rotation. We used the TPRT to release his internal hip rotators and then built strength with the Bosch Activation: Half Moon. As you can see, he now has a full 40° of hip internal rotation. This type of therapy improved his joint mobility, helping him move in the lateral plane when hitting his forehand.

HIP EXTERNAL ROTATORS- QUADRATUS FEMORIS – SMALL KNOB & FLAT EDGE

LUBRICATION: None

TPRT:

Small Knob

TECHNIQUE MOTION:

1 - Assess External Hip Rotation. How many degrees do they have out of 90°?

2 - Palpate the lateral Trochanter with your fingers

3 - Place the Flat Edge of the TPRT on the Quadratus Femoris. Have the client breathe in for 3 seconds, then move up and down (distal proximal) and side to side (lateral/medial) as they exhale.

4 - Place the knob of the TPRT on the Quadratus Femoris. Use your left hand to move the knob distal or lateral from the Trochanter.

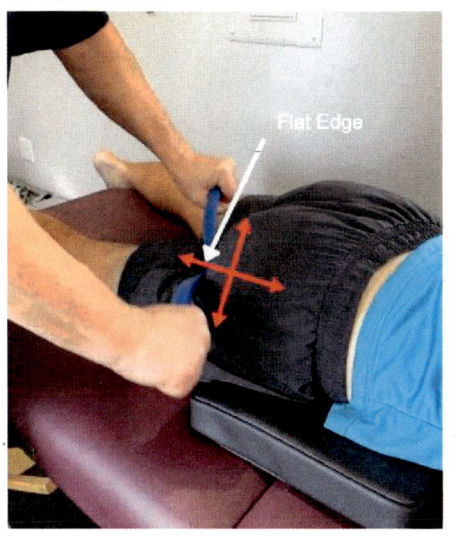

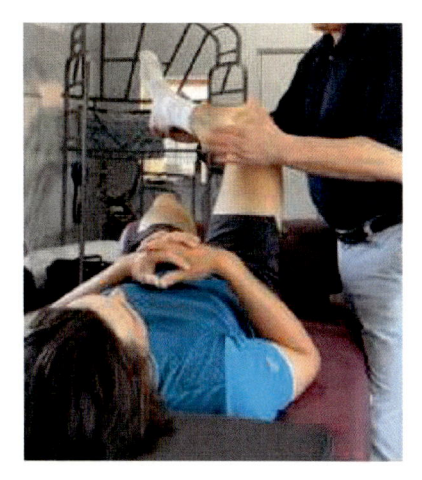

Hip Ext Rotation Range of Motion Assessment

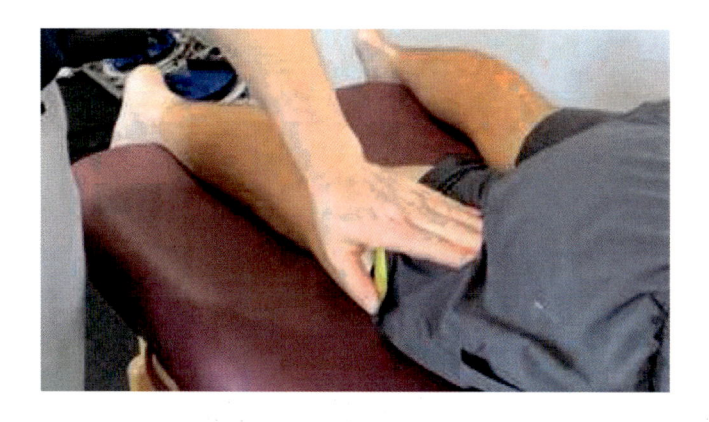

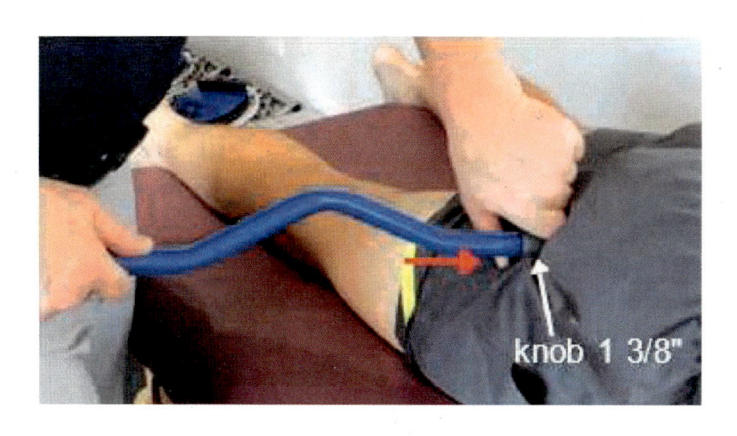

QUADRATUS LUMBORUM (SIDELYING) – V & CURVES

LUBRICATION: Oil or Lotion

TPRT:
Curves and V

TECHNIQUE MOTION:

Have the client lie on their side. Place lotion on the lower back. Place the Curves, and the V just superior to the ilium. Lightly work up and away from the ilium.

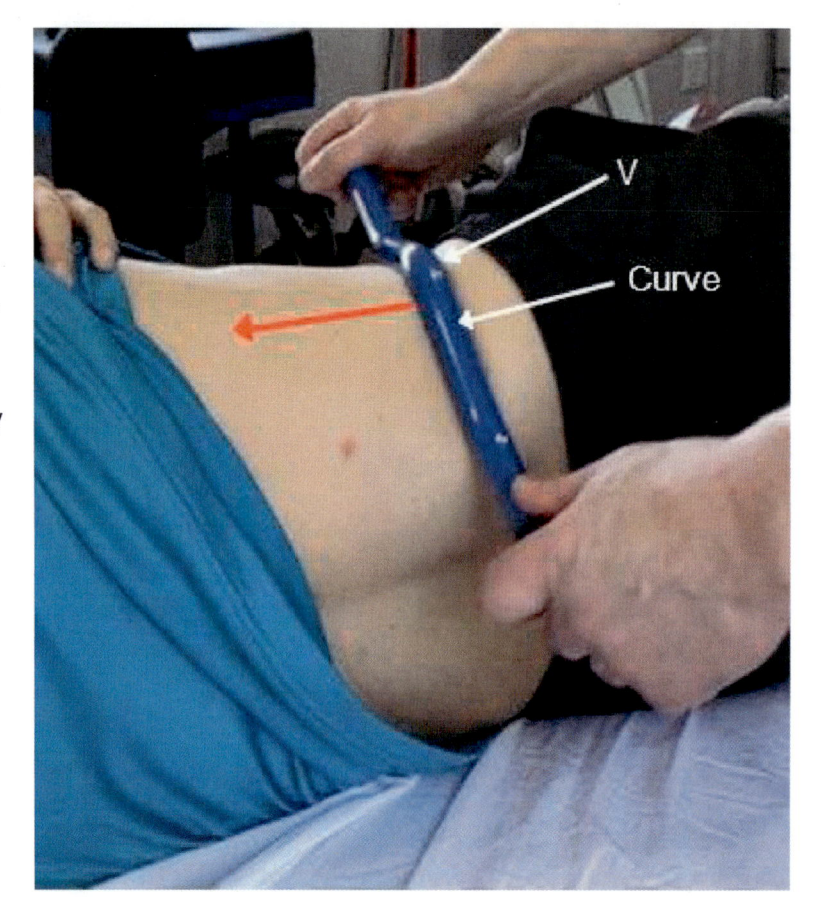

Quadratus Lumborum – Curves, V

LATISSIMUS DORSI (PRONE) – SLOPE & CURVE

LUBRICATION: None

TPRT:
Curve and Slope

TECHNIQUE MOTION:
Place the Slope on the latissimus dorsi attachment just above the ilium.

Stay off the bone and pivot the TPRT lightly back and forth (Like a seesaw).

Note: Be sure to stay off the kidneys.

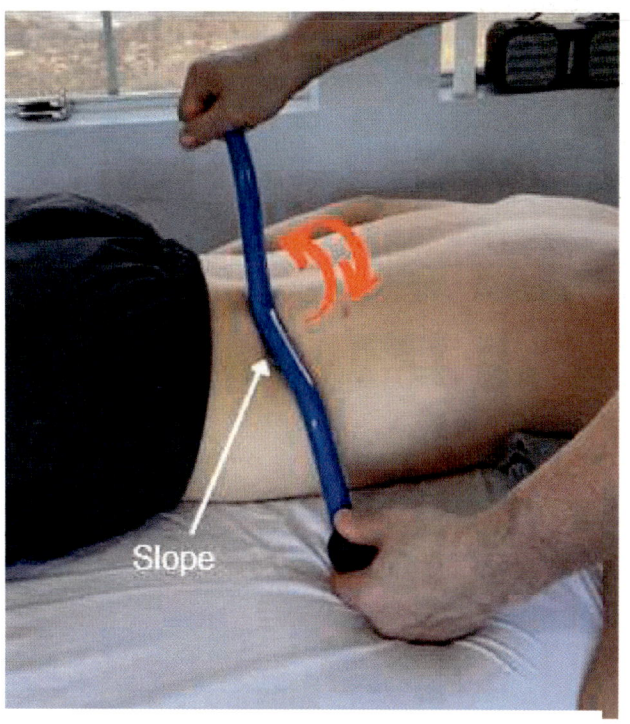

Latissimus Dorsi – Slope

BACK RELEASE (PRONE) - SMALL KNOB

LUBRICATION: None

TPRT:
Small Knob

TECHNIQUE MOTION:
Place the knob on the Longissimus Thoracis.

Move the knob from <u>inferior to superior and superior to inferior</u>, and also work in a <u>circular motion</u>.

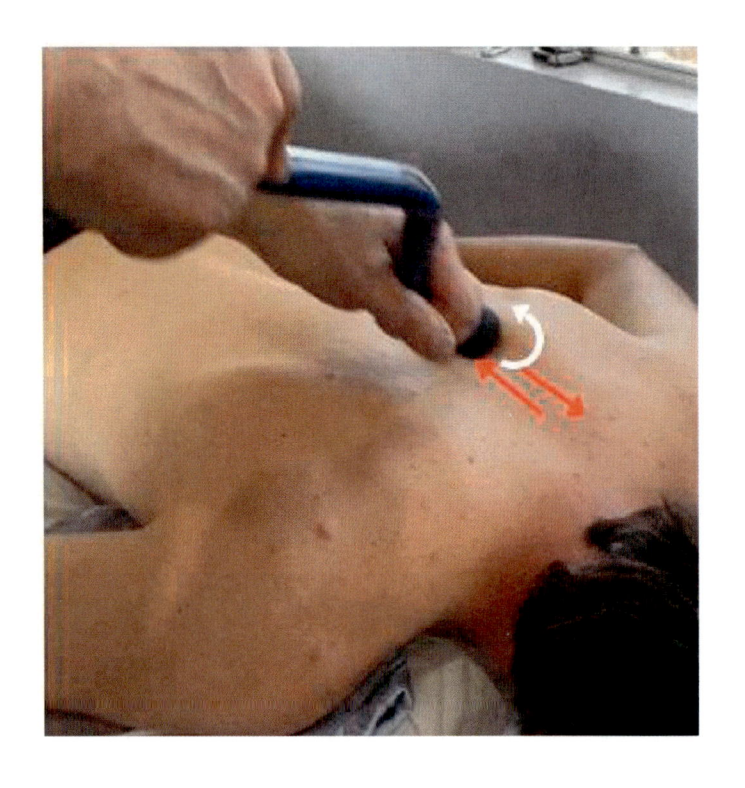

Back Release – Small Knob

BACK RELEASE (SEATED) - SMALL KNOB

LUBRICATION: None

TPRT:
Small Knob

TECHNIQUE MOTION:
Have the client place their hand on the opposite shoulder from the side you are working on.

Place the knob just lateral to the spine. Engage the Traps with the knob and work laterally away from the spine. Also, work superior and inferior and work in a circular motion.

Have the client breathe in for 3 seconds, then exhale as you apply pressure. Repeat 2 to 3 times or until the trigger point releases. Then, move to another spot and repeat.

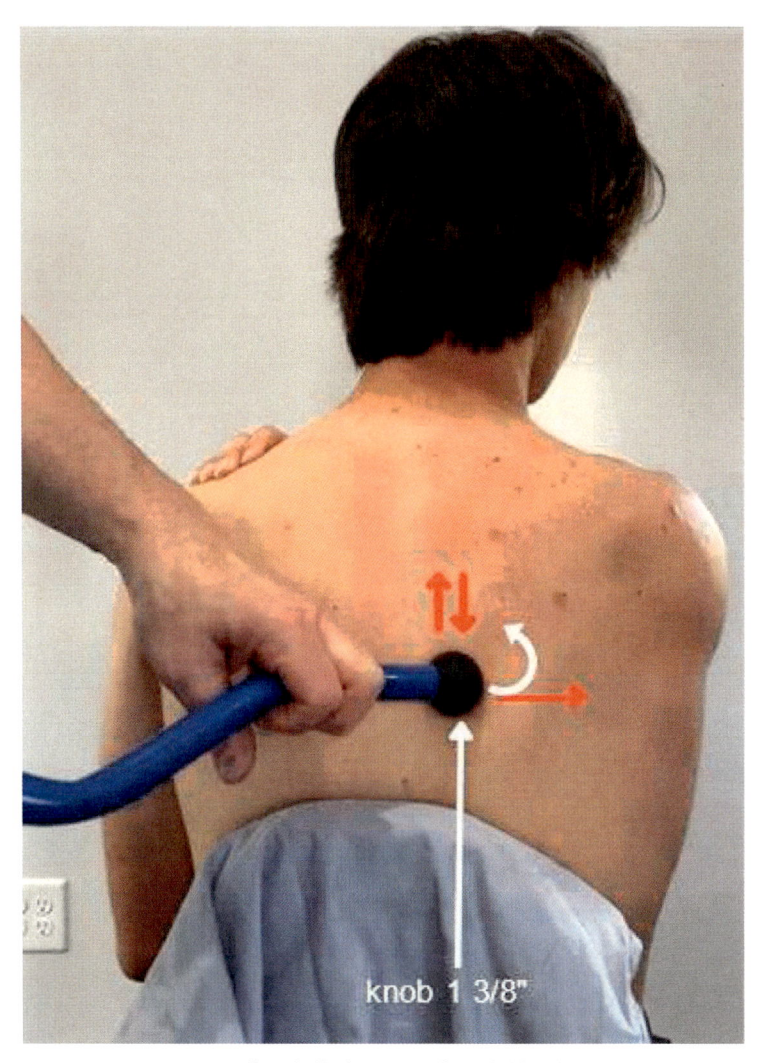

Back Release – Small Knob

TPRT MODULE 7 – CLIENT THERAPY

TRAP RELEASE (SEATED) - CURVE

LUBRICATION: Lotion

TPRT:
Curve

TECHNIQUE MOTION:
Place the Curve on the traps and <u>slide</u> up into the neck.

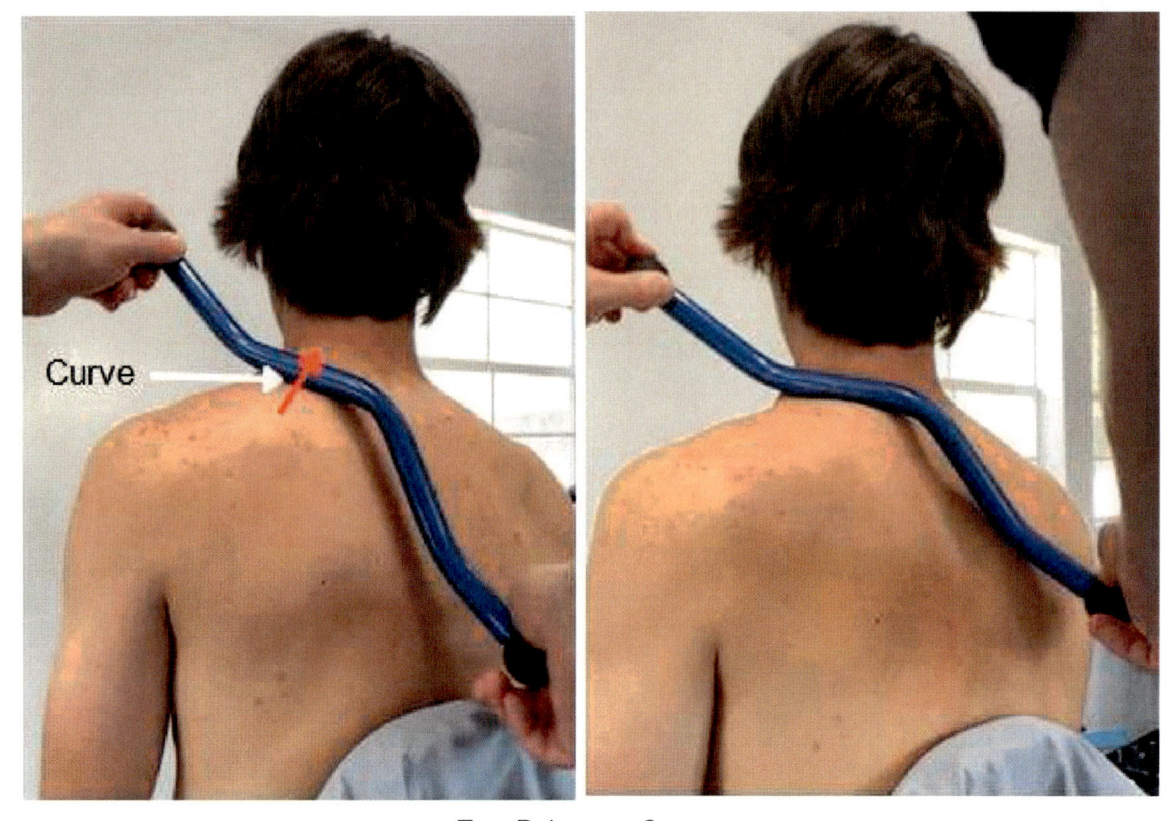

Trap Release – Curve

LOWER BACK RELEASE (STANDING) - CURVE

LUBRICATION: Lotion

TPRT:
Curve

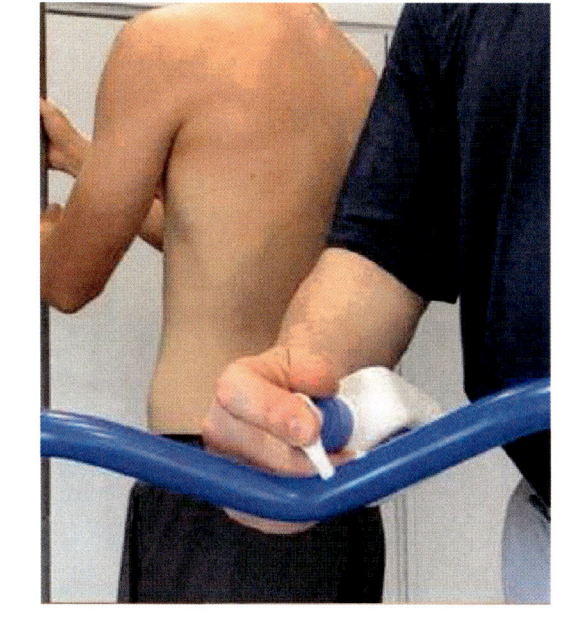

TECHNIQUE MOTION:
Apply lotion to the TPRT and on the lower back.

Place the Curve just above the ilium and slide in the superior and inferior directions (up and down).

Avoid direct contact over the kidneys. Do not use the TPRT to pivot over the kidneys with the knobs, Flat Edges, or Points.

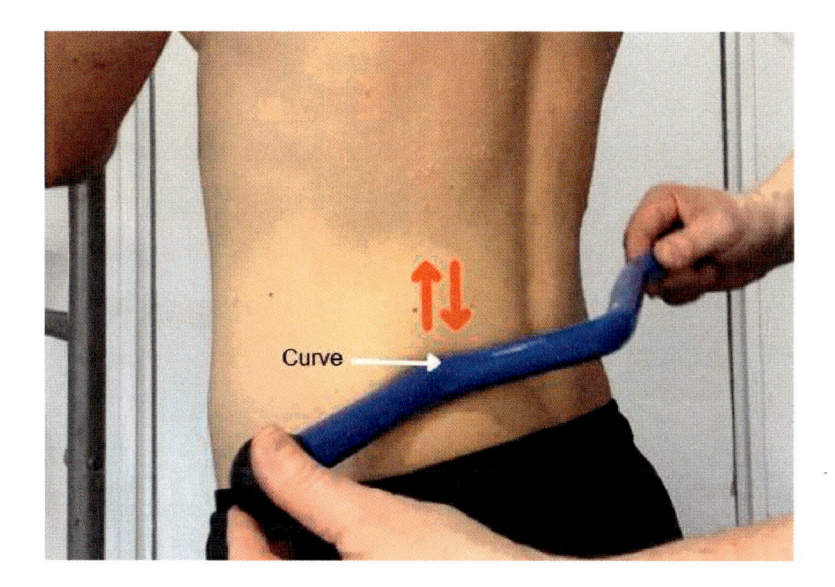

RECTUS ABDOMINIS AND INTERNAL OBLIQUE RELEASE – SLOPE

LUBRICATION: Lotion

TPRT:
Slope

TECHNIQUE MOTION:
Put lotion on the abs and obliques.

Place the Slope just inferior to the ribs. <u>Slide</u> the TPRT down the abs to the pubic bone.

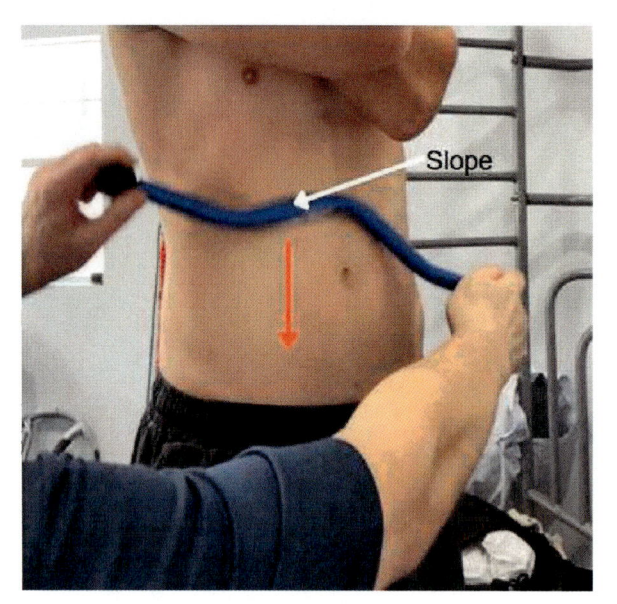

Abs & Obliques Release– Slope

SOME OF GREG'S CLIENTS

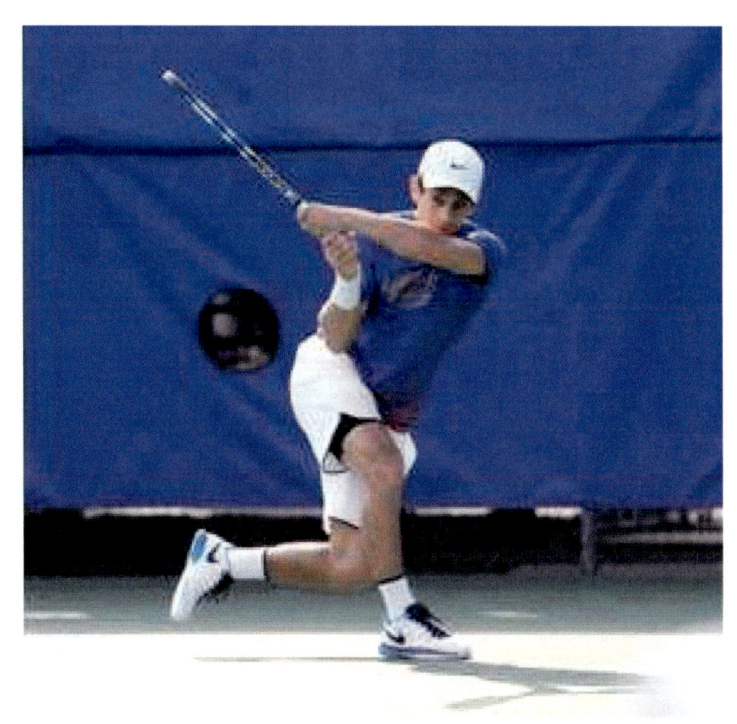

Elliot Orkin - Tennis player who went to the University of Florida and worked with Greg.

Greg's colleagues from the Tennis Team at the University of South Carolina (From L-R):

Asst. Coach; Ryan Young, Player; Thomas Mayronne, Head coach; Josh Goffi, Player; Harrison O'Keefe

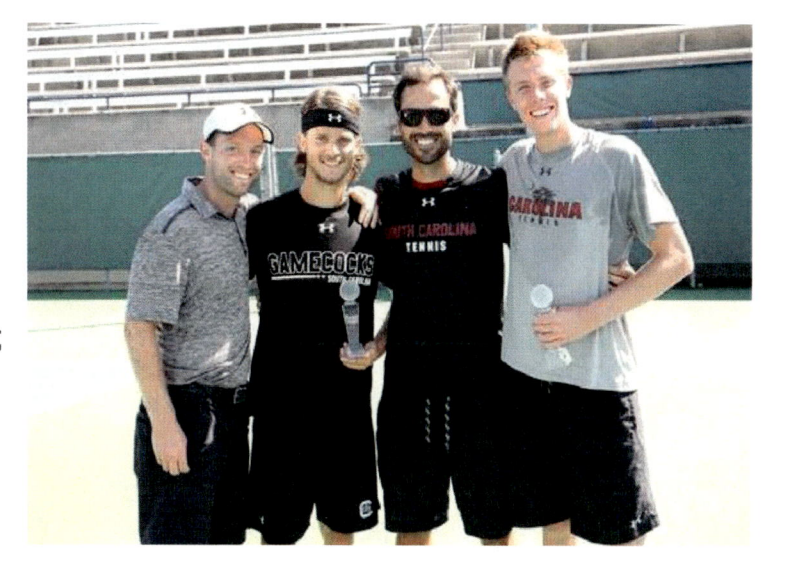

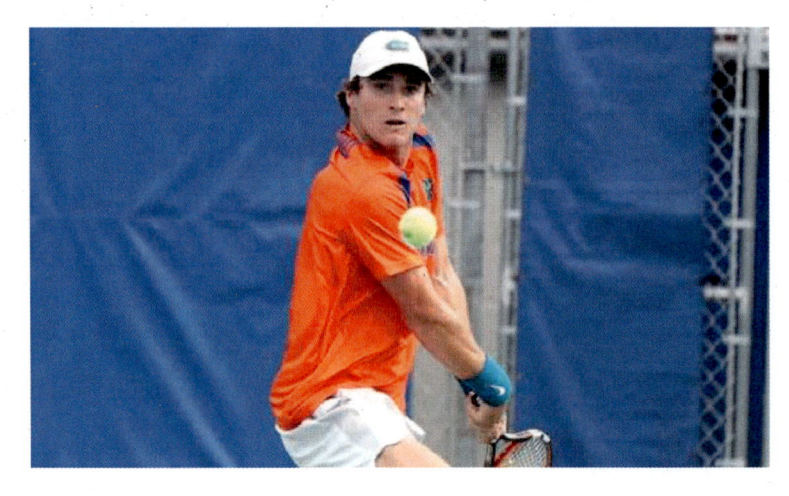

Oliver Crawford - Pro. Tennis Player (Current ATP Ranking - 215) who works with Greg.

Marianna Singletary - Volleyball Player for the University of Texas 2023 NCAA Volleyball Champions

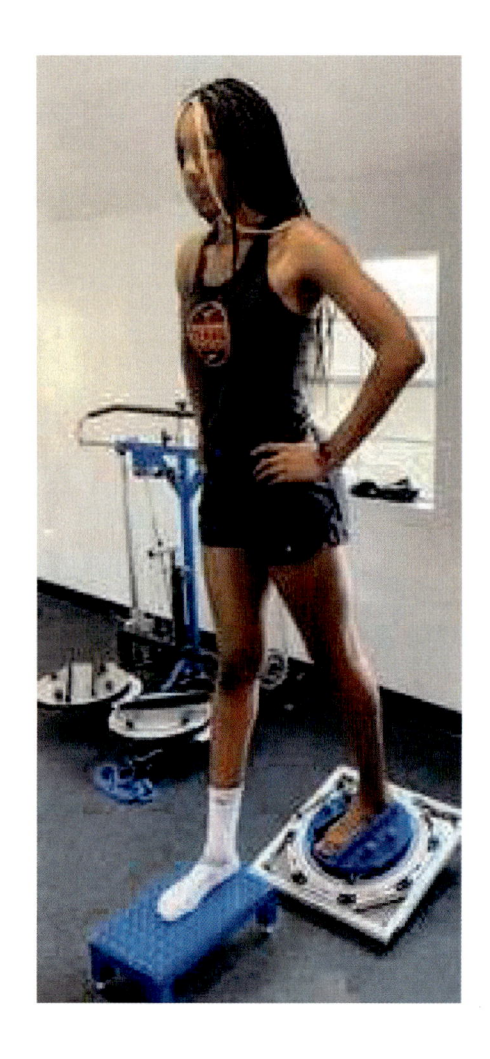

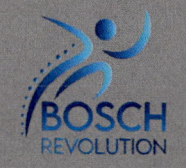

CONCLUSION

In these pages, you learned about the Trigger Point Release Tool™ and all its indications and contraindications. You also learned how many people can safely and effectively use it to help themselves and clients in various ways by adding it to other training modalities such as CrossFit, cycling, running, weight training, yoga, and Pilates.

Important Links and Resources to continue your journey:

https://www.kenthealth.com/safety-protocols-the-carotid-artery/

https://www.kenthealth.com/posture-chart-forward-head-posture/

https://www.kenthealth.com/trigger-point-chart-pain-management- without-opioids/

https://www.nature.com/articles/s41598-021-92194-z

As this book closes, I hope it leaves you with a profound understanding of the indispensable role that proper muscle and fascia care play in maintaining an active, injury-free lifestyle. Whether you are an athlete striving for peak performance, a weekend warrior, or someone navigating the daily challenges of physical wellness, the techniques and tools discussed here are designed to enhance your muscular health and overall well-being. The journey to optimum physical health is continuous and evolving, and with the Trigger Point Release Tool™ at your disposal, you are well-equipped to face this journey head-on. Remember, the key to movement is not just motion, but mindful, informed, and healthy practices that sustain and enrich your life's activities.

To connect with me for more, to purchase other materials, book a session, or attend one of my seminars, please visit https://boschrevolution.com.

Thank you for joining me on this path to better health and heightened body awareness.

Made in United States
Orlando, FL
27 June 2024